THE HEALTHY HAIRSTYLIST

DR. JONAS EYFORD

ISBN:978-0-9950902-1-7

Hɛːstʌɪlɪst

CONTENTS

ABOUT THIS BOOK

Opening with thoughts on understanding your body, this book outlines the best and worst working habits, profiles a range of relevant conditions, their causes and treatment options. Earlier chapters contain practical advice and simple strategies to improve your general condition. A few chapters cover specific issues, steps to take to recover, pain and adapt your behavior. Later chapters cover skin and respiratory health, techniques to improve sleep and overall physical condition.

Sections relevant to all salon workers

Body Awareness

Understanding the Strains

Optimal Biomechanics

Choosing Good Footwear

Pain & How to Fix It

Preventative Exercise

Sleep

Skin Health

Respiratory Health

Sections best used for specific issues

Common Mistakes

Specific Injuries & Conditions

Helpful Tools & Resources

Appendix

5-minute plans

Exercise Appendix

INTRODUCTION

This book is meant to help hairstylists improve their health and better withstand the physical strains involved in their work.

Working as a hairstylist involves a lot of repetitive movements and straining postures. This puts great physical demands on hairstylists which can lead to pain in the neck, shoulder, wrist and hand, feet and back. Throughout the industry there is a lack of support for those dealing with health issues and a general lack of guidelines for best ergonomic practices. This book is meant to help hairstylists improve their health and better withstand the physical strains involved in their work. I have treated hundreds of hairstylists in my chiropractic practice over the years, and worked with hundreds more researching and consulting at salons across the country. When I started seeing a lot of hairstylists I noticed two things: that certain problems are very common, and that no matter how well we would fix them, they would often be back after a couple months. Prevention and self-management of health issues seem to be the key to thriving as a hairstylist. Staying healthy requires an understanding of how your work habits affect your body, but also a desire to improve. By taking care of your body, you can do more than just prevent repetitive strain injuries; you can enhance energy levels, performance, efficiency, mood and by extension you can catalyze financial success and career longevity. A focused effort on simple changes can yield powerful results. This book is full of simple changes and practical techniques from a robust set of experience that can yield marked improvement in your health and capacity to perform. Each time we make a small decision that improves our health, we feel better, which in turn makes it easier to continue making great choices. This book aims to improve the quality of life for hairstylists everywhere.

1

Body Awareness

"The body never lies."
- Martha Graham

BODY AWARENESS

Your body is the most complex piece of technology you will ever control. Above all it is important to understand that it thrives in moderation. Strive for balance and learn to listen to your body. Becoming more aware of how your body works and what you are doing to your body while at work is the crucial first step to enhancing your physical well-being. The stresses on your body as a hairstylist are numerous. Certain parts of your body are worked excessively.

When the demands on your body exceed its ability to sustain them, your body speaks to you. Pain is your body's way of telling you something is wrong. NEVER ignore pain. Take the time to interpret the signal and think for a moment about why you are feeling pain. If you suspect your body is in pain because you've worked it too hard, you must first reverse the effects of the strain (rest, postural changes, stretches, therapies, assistive devices) and then strengthen your body until you can tolerate more of that activity (exercise). This book will help you through each step of the process of dealing with injury, identifying the cause of pain, correcting the problem, and then enhancing your body's capacity.

If you are experiencing pain frequently, start taking notes. At the end of each day, jot down five things:

1 Where you felt pain

2 When you felt it

3 What you were doing immediately before or while you felt it (standing, bending, blow drying, shampooing, highlights, etc.)

4 The character of the pain (sharp, dull, stabbing, burning, achy, deep, etc.)

5 What made it feel better (resting, stretching, heat, ice, pain-killers, etc.)

BENEFITS OF TAKING NOTES

Taking notes for days or weeks at a time will help you in three ways. It will help you notice patterns, it will help you better recognize the nature of the problem when cross-referencing your issue with the descriptions of conditions later in this book, and it will help your health care practitioner properly diagnose your condition if you seek help. It is important to become aware of the strains your work places on your body, and learn how to deal with them before they become chronic issues. Once you are aware of the problem it is easier to know how to minimize the strain, treat the damage and prevent further strain. One study done on hairstylists in Brazil found that the biggest risk factor for musculoskeletal disorders was not acknowledging the strains associated with work.[1] Simply acknowledging the risks of your work proved to be more important for well-being than how long you've been working and more important than discomfort felt while working. If you are still reading this, you have already taken the first big step to having a healthy and pain-free body.

BENEFITS OF STANDING AT WORK

It is worth mentioning that compared to the majority of the population, the physical benefits of the type of work you do are significant. The simple fact that you spend most the day standing and moving around is more beneficial than you may think. The increased amount of movement contributes to the health of your joints and your general health. It's important to capitalize on this advantage, just as it's important to neutralize the type of work that is tough on your body. Ensuring proper posture for instance is one way of capitalizing. More than just preventing injury and strain, good working postures will encourage the development of muscles and keep your spine, bones and joints healthy. Wearing supportive footwear, balancing and varying your activities, and eating well are also examples of ways you can ensure that time spent at work is productive to your health.

1. Gisele Mussi and Nelson Gouveia, "Prevalence of Work-Related Musculoskeletal Disorders in Brazilian Hairdressers," Occupational Medicine 58 (2008)

Understanding the Strains

"The part can never be well unless the whole is well."
- Plato

UNDERSTANDING THE STRAINS

Pain is a signal from your body tissues to your brain telling you something is wrong. Never ignore pain. Rather than just coping with pain killers, practice listening to what your body is telling you to get a sense of what you need to heal. To do this we need to understand a little about what might be happening in our bodies when we experience pain.

Pain is often the result of inflammation. Inflammation serves to protect your body when it is injured. Like airbags protecting you in a car crash, the process of inflammation protects the damaged area from further injury and attracts repair cells to the region, serving as the important first step in tissue repair.

After working for hours, standing with your back arched too much, bending forward too often, or leaning on one hip too frequently, inflammation can start to accumulate. The only way to prevent this type of strain is to improve postures and to move with more diversity. Even *with* good posture, holding any one position for an extended period of time can be detrimental. This is because prolonged static contractions of muscle reduces the blood flow to the area and cramps nearby joints. With reduced blood flow and tense muscles, your joints are more likely to become inflamed and painful, lose their range of motion and eventually degenerate sooner than they should. Practically, this entails that we should break up our repetitive postures using diverse movements as much as possible.

It is useful to differentiate between the two purposes of muscle activation: movement and stabilization. Generally, the larger muscles of your body move joints and the smaller muscles stabilize them. Without specific guidance, we are always inclined to move our bodies with just the completion of a task in mind. We are wired to move efficiently, which is great. However, when we are required to perform certain movements over and over again, it is then important to re-train the movement to be safe as well as efficient. If we want to preserve the integrity of the tissues and joints in our bodies we must learn to move in ways that optimize the activation of the smaller, weaker stabilization muscles. The shortcut to figuring out how to position your body to move safely is to pretend that you are holding something that weighs a lot. When you are preparing to move something heavy, your nervous system kicks up a gear and fires more muscles. This mental trick is useful when working on improving postures and reducing pain.

The movement optimization techniques in this book serve to help you identify dysfunctional movement and reorganize it to improve the sustainability of the most common of your movements at work.

SHOULDER

The most important factor in terms of shoulder health for hairstylists is the position of the shoulder blade while the arms are elevated. The shoulder blades should be held back and together to maintain the space for shoulder muscles to glide. When the arms are reaching forward and the shoulder blades slide forward, the

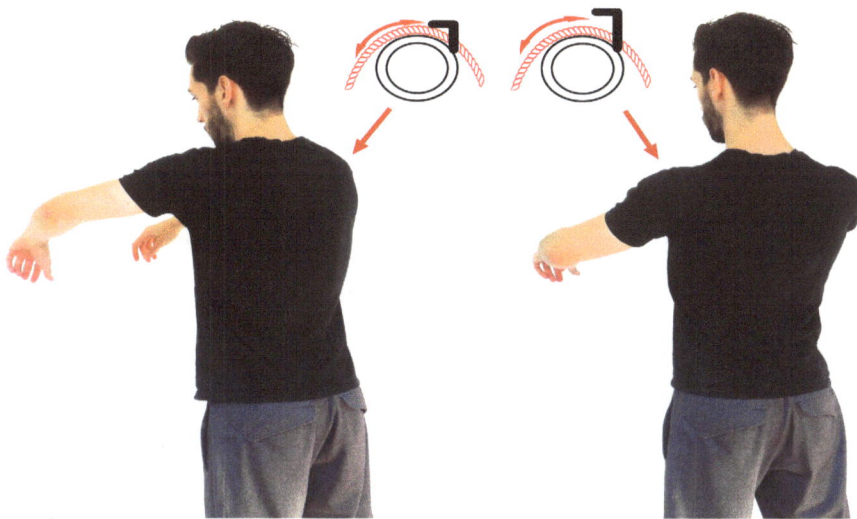

Demonstrating bad versus good shoulder position

space for the rotator cuff muscles to move through shrinks and can lead to premature fraying of the tendons. When this happens it's called shoulder impingement. It's quite common among hairstylists and it's very preventable.

Improving the shoulder blade position will also re-arrange the way your muscles are being used. Proper shoulder blade posture (together and down) facilitates more activation of your larger back, shoulder and arm muscles and spares the more delicate rotator cuff muscles. It will also help to reduce the amount of wear and tear of the three main joints of the shoulder – the glenohumeral joint, the sternoclavicular joint and the acromioclavicular joint.

The image above compares the anatomy of the shoulder to a pulley system to help illustrate the impact of shoulder blade position. The rope represents the supraspinatus muscle (the rotator cuff muscle most injured among hairstylists) and the narrowing space represents the acromiohumeral joint space. The further your shoulder blades drift forward, the smaller the space is for the supraspinatus to move through and the higher your chances of developing shoulder impingement and pain. Thus the importance of working on keeping your shoulder blades back and down.

NECK

The neck should spend most of its time in a neutral position at the top of the spine. A weak neck tends to migrate forwards, which causes excess strain on the posterior neck muscles and encourages slouching. The head weighs about 11 pounds. The graphic on the next page uses some physics to demonstrate how extensive the effects of poor neck posture can be. It shows how tilting your head forward 8 inches places increased force (5 lbs) through the tiny set of muscles in the

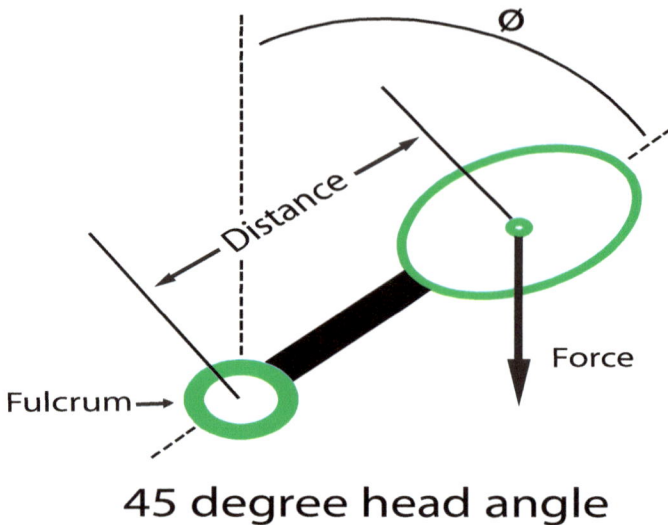

Ø = 45 degrees

Force = 11 pounds

Distance = 8 inches

Torque = Force x distance to fulcrum x sin of ø

Torque = 11 lbs x 0.66 ft x sin45
= 11 x 0.66 x 0.71
= 5.15 foot pounds
= 6.98 Newton meters

45 degree head angle

Calculation showing how holding your head forward several inches is like holding up a 7 pound weight

back of your neck. Imagine how difficult it would be to hold up a 5lb weight in your hand for hours at a time. If you are like most hairstylists, always carrying a lot of tension in the back of the neck, you will want to work on reducing it using better postural techniques that you'll find in the next chapter.

LOW BACK

Standing (uninterrupted) for long periods of time in the same positions certainly strains your body, your low back in particular. It can also be hard on your feet, ankles, knees and hips. It is valuable to remember that your body thrives with diversity of movement. The more movement the better - as long as the activity and type of movement varies. Think about how you can walk a lot longer without discomfort than

you can stand still. The challenge for hairstylists is the demand of performing the same activities many times over, day after day. Any effort to break up the repetition of your activities or modify the way you perform them is an effort that will contribute to your physical well-being. Try your best to organize your schedule in ways that will help prevent excessive repetition. It's a thought easily dismissed by the busy stylist, but remember that the cumulative effects of small changes can be significant. Blow drys (hard on the shoulders and wrists) or childrens cuts (hard on the low back) for instance should be spread apart as much as possible. To neglect your body's needs in favor of your duties is only selling short your ability to do your best work for a longer time. It's much more difficult to recover from an injury than to make the small changes to prevent one. It helps to be vocal about your priority of staying healthy. Help your coworkers understand why you want to make the small changes to the organization of your day. When it's too difficult to re-arrange the schedule, it is very manageable to take on a few stretches and exercises that offset the specific strains you experience at work. You can integrate them into your day or do them at the end of a day. You'll find useful specific suggestions in the Pain and How to Fit It chapter.

The low back is a complex area, managing pain or discomfort is best done by first understanding how your work affects it, increasing awareness of postural and movement habits and then practicing the self-treatment techniques explored later in this book.

Chronic low back pain is typically the result of either a lack of movement or too much of one kind of movement. Standing is not harmful to your low back on its own, even for long periods of time, provided that you have developed the muscular endurance necessary to support your spine for longer durations. Only reasonable levels of core endurance are needed if we ensure a diversity of movement

The fact that you spend a significant amount of time standing throughout the day is in fact a huge advantage you have over all the unfortunate people stuck in an office chair all day. It is well established in the research that people performing jobs with heavy repetitive movements (nurses, factory workers) are the most susceptible to back pain, followed by workers who sit for most of the day (office workers, truck drivers). Research consistently reinforces the notion that both sitting and standing uninterrupted for extended periods of time are bad for the low back and for overall health.

There are three scientific concepts that can help us better understand the common causes of low back pain. The first is the effect of compression, the second is CREEP and the third is deconditioning.

Compression. Our spines and our core muscles serve as the shock absorbers of our body. The curves of our spine increase its ability to absorb shock, and the large curve of the low back bears the brunt of compressive forces. Throughout the day, the combined compressive forces of gravity and of muscle contraction compact our spine. The position of our torso heavily influences the extent of forces that transfer through our low back. The more endurance our core muscles have, the more able we are to maintain optimal spinal posture and reduce the impact of compression, as depicted below.

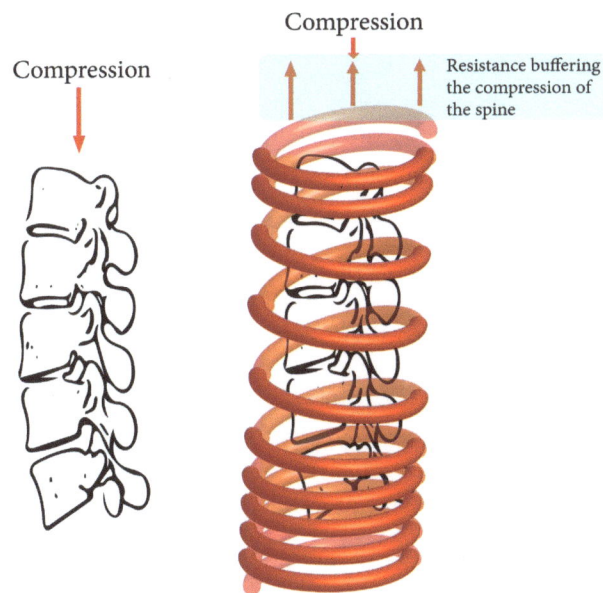

Compression

Compression

Resistance buffering the compression of the spine

Core muscles lessen compression on the spine

Our sleeping habits also have an impact on the integrity of our spines. The intervertebral discs (the discs between each of the spinal vertebrae) are slowly drained of some of their fluid throughout the day and are replenished at night while we sleep.

Considering this relationship between abdominals and the spine a little further, it helps to acknowledge how every movement has a counter movement which transmits compressive forces through the spine. For example, if I am standing and reach my right arm forward to shake someone's hand, the momentum of my arm moving forward is countered by the opposite part of the body - the lower left part of my torso and pelvis in this case. The forces caused by the muscle contractions are transmitted through my body, mostly through the low back and pelvis. The low back serves as the fulcrum that buffers forces between the upper and lower body, the left and the right side. This means that virtually every movement of your body - even those not including any bending - involve (and can potentially strain) the low back. This is a useful concept to understand because if you want to improve the amount of time you can work without back pain, you have to know to work on more than just your standing posture; you'll want to improve your posture through reaching, pulling, pushing and bending movements too. Through these movements, the more active and strong your core, pelvic and thigh muscles are, the less forces are transmitted through the joints of your low back.

CREEP stands for Continuous Repetitive Elongation of the Elastic Properties of tissue. If you keep your body in a certain position for extended periods of time, the tissue begins to lose its elasticity. This is why extensive sitting is so harmful; it stretches out all the tendons, ligaments, muscles and fascia of the low back region. CREEP sets in after as little as 10-15 minutes. Tissues need to move frequently, and move into the opposite of the position that it spends the most time in. If you stand upright for hours on end, the best things you can do for a break are stretch the short & tight muscles, relax the overused muscles (sit or lie down) or anything active that has you moving differently from the positions you maintain while working.

Deconditioning is the gradual loss of strength in a muscle group when it is used improperly or not enough. We can consider the muscles of the low back to be in two groups: movers or stabilizers. The movers are the big strong muscles that twist and bend you. They rarely become deconditioned. The stabilizers on the other hand are prone to becoming deconditioned. They are the small muscles situated deeper down, close to the spine, that have the important job of fine-tuning movements of your joints as the movers move them. This is an incredibly important job when it comes to the spine and particularly the low back. When we sit, the stabilizer muscles turn off. When our posture is poor our stabilizers are turned down. And when our stabilizers are constantly turned down or turned off, they become weak and deconditioned. Once deconditioned, you are more susceptible to strains and injuries because the joints start to move in suboptimal ways, wearing down cartilage and straining ligaments. If your back gets sore relatively quickly or you frequently 'throw out' your back, you probably have weak stabilizer muscles. Through my clinical experience, I have found that hairstylists who exercise regularly are far less likely to have pain related to muscle fatigue. Exercise or activities of any variety can improve physical endurance and prevent pain; anything from yoga and pilates to running, weight lifting, swimming or sports of any kind.

A very important stabilizer muscle in the low back is called the multifidus. If you train this muscle to be more active, not only will you strain your back less often, you will be able to stand and work longer without getting sore.

If you suffer from back pain in a specific area (it can be considered specific if you can put your finger on the pain), refer to the section on Pain and How to Fix It.

If you suffer from general soreness throughout your low back when you work, you will benefit from the next chapter on Optimal Biomechanics.

It is important to listen to your body, understand what is happening when you feel pain, and to take a proactive approach to dealing with it. Your general approach to managing pain and strain should include diversifying your activities and improving the posture with which you perform straining tasks.

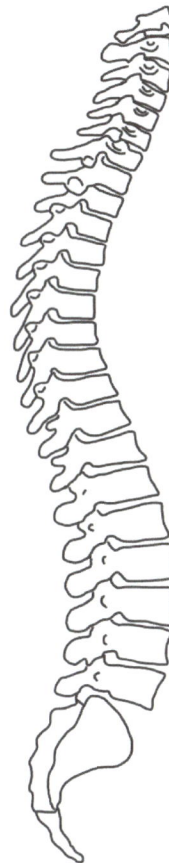

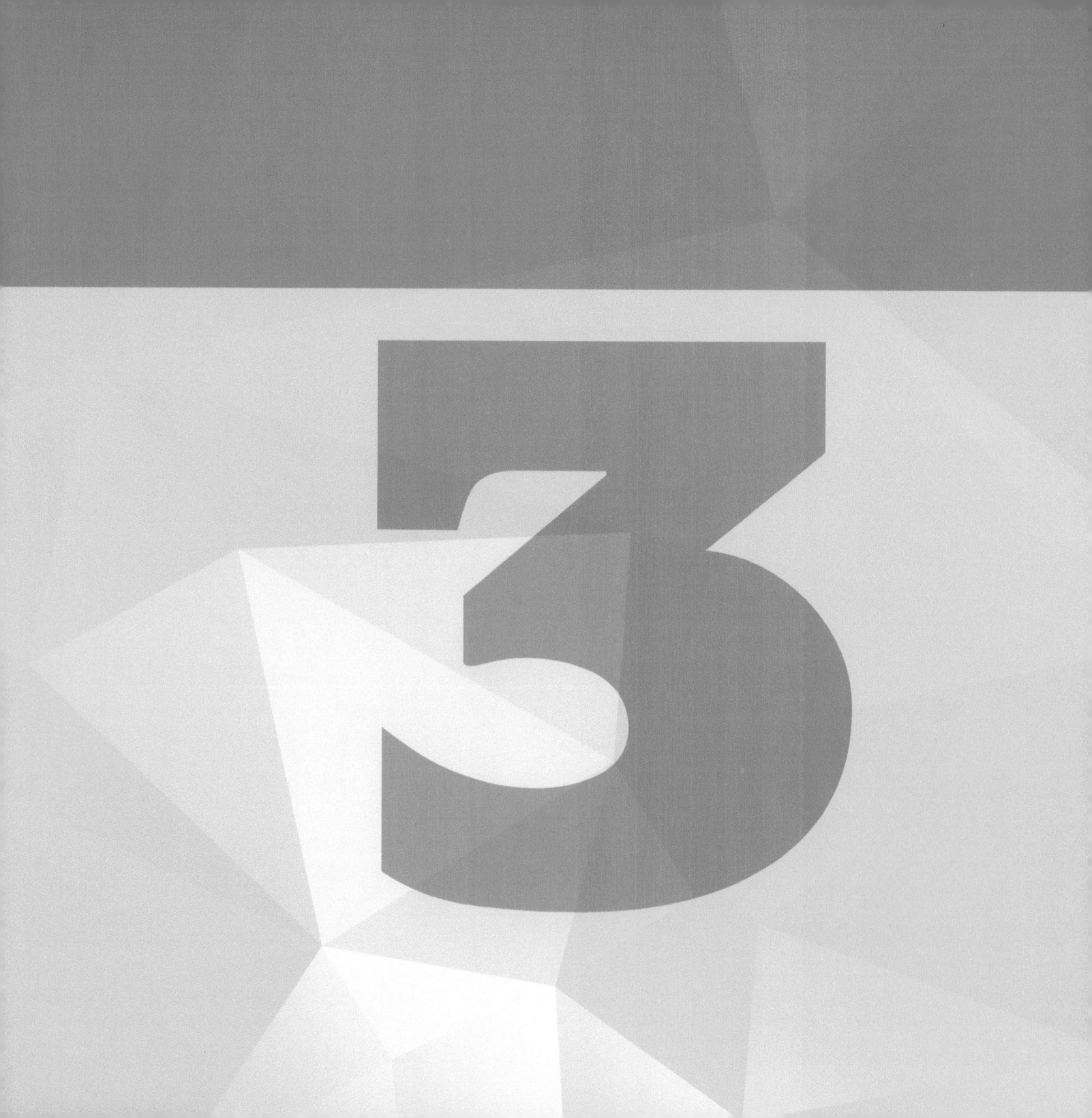

3

Optimal Biomechanics

"There is more wisdom in your body than in your deepest philosophies."
- Friedrich Nietzche

OPTIMAL BIOMECHANICS

The techniques you must employ to ensure that your body maintains optimal positions throughout the day are relatively easy to grasp but tough to master. Like any form of physical activity, it takes time and discipline to develop. Be patient to reap the benefits.

Make your activities harder to make your life easier. It is a simple but powerful concept. Let's explore a simple example; you drop your comb. Your natural inclination is to reach down by bending your low back while keeping your legs strait. The much better option is to bend mostly at the hips and a little at the knees, keeping your back relatively strait. We subconsciously choose the first option because it is the most energy efficient. Our bodies are designed to be efficient, which is great in many ways but it compromises our (long term) safety when we perform activities repetitively. This is where our conscious mind comes in. We must override our inclination for quick easy movements in favor of more responsible movements in order to preserve the integrity of our bodies over time. The more you invest in developing robust movement habits, the more of a buffer you will have between health and injury. A good tip is to imagine the comb (or whatever you want to pick up) is A LOT heavier than it really is. This triggers your nervous system to fire up more muscles and lift in a much more responsible way.

The two most important elements of your standing posture are your shoulder blade posture and the way you use your hips and pelvis.

IMPROVING UPPER BODY POSTURE

Stand upright with both hands on your chest. Hold your elbows behind your shoulders and your chin behind your hands.

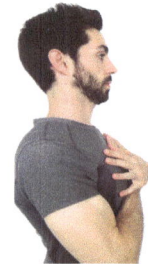

Once you have set your ideal upper body position, holding your shoulder blades together and down while you use your arms will maintain it. This activates larger torso muscles, taking the strain off the smaller shoulder muscles. It also significantly increases the space in the shoulder joint for tendons and muscles to move around.

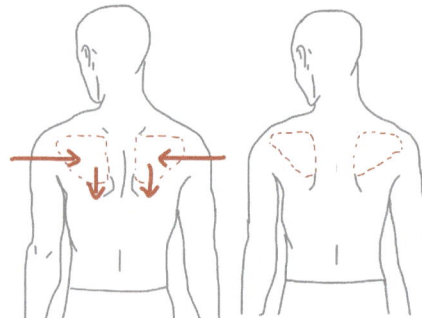

Two things happen when your shoulder is in the unsafe position; the rotator cuff muscles are stretched while they work, and the shoulder joint sits in a compromised position, compressing the supraspinatus tendon. Prolonged use of the arm in this position will wear out acromioclavicular joint and the supraspinatus tendon rather quickly.

Corrective exercises for shoulder problems are found in the chapter on specific injuries and conditions.

To really master good working shoulder posture, it can be very helpful to use postural kinesiology tape, elastic postural braces, strengthening exercises for the upper back muscles, and a posture buddy at work (someone who keeps their eye on you and reminds you to improve your posture when you are slacking off). In most cases, excessively tight muscles will impede progress. A therapist (massage, sports therapist, chiropractor, physiotherapist) can help resolve built up muscle tension.

IMPROVING LOWER BODY POSTURE

The key to good lower body posture is using gluteal and abdominal muscles optimally.

This will produce a healthy, safe neutral spinal position and significantly reduce the strain on your spine.

Increasing the activation of your abdominals increases the compressive forces going through your lower back. Activating your gluteal muscles ensures that you're using your strongest muscles to keep you upright, reducing the forces going through your joints reducing the chances of developing back pain when standing for extended periods of time.

To activate your gluteal muscles, squeeze your buttocks together, do a Kegel contraction, pull your ribcage down vertically, harden your abdominals and make sure your ears are in line with your shoulders.

Practicing good posture is the first step. The next is to learn how to move well.

MOVE AT THE HIPS

Perhaps the most important change a hairstylist with back pain can make is increasing the use of hips and knees during regular movements. Doing so around the client will spare your back and neck while also strengthening your legs. It takes a lot of work to develop the habit and to build the strength to move with your hips consistently, but can spare you years of pain and problems; well worth the effort if you ask me.

When bending over, bend your knees only slightly, keep your low back arched and hinge up and down through your hips. Increasing the amount of forward bending movement happens at your hips is an immensely productive habit to practice.

Practice tilting your pelvis slightly forwards and

backwards and teach yourself to sway gently from side to side instead of leaning on one hip. Leaning on your hip to one side is a lazy stance that has negative effects on the alignment of the whole body.

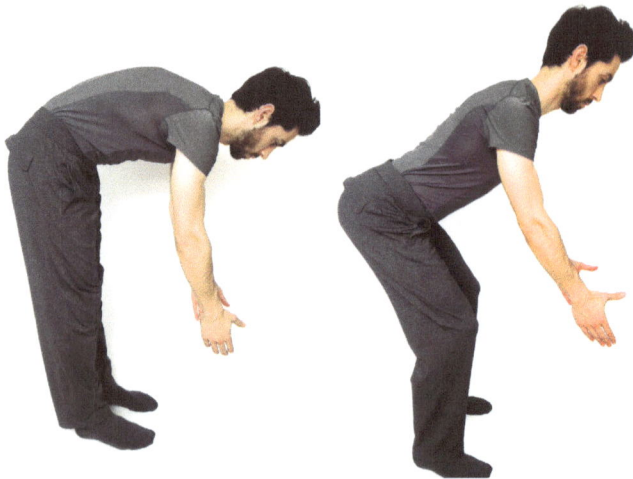

BAD   **GOOD**

It is helpful to stand with your feet in an offset position. It allows for more movement, increases the activation of pelvic and gluteal muscles and decreases strain put on the back (both upper and lower). Try not to favor one side, alternate back and forth.

A really good tip for those who get a sore back after standing all day, is to constantly change the position of your low back. Holding an abdominal contraction is

only sustainable for several minutes at a time. It takes a lot of work to improve your abdominal endurance so it is important to know that having good posture is not 'all or nothing'. Slowly rotating your pelvis forwards and backwards and tilting side to side provides the constant movement your body craves. It sounds really simple, and it is! Take it seriously, make small efforts to move more consistently and it will make a difference. Keeping your lower back in any one position for too long it will stress the tissue and cause pain. Take any chance you have throughout the day to do a little stretching. Even 5 second stretches done sporadically throughout the day can serve to reduce the cumulative strain of working postures. Many hairstylists stay out of pain by doing subtle exercises and stretches while working (slow calf raises, shallow lunges or abdominal contractions for instance). Low back pain can often be complex, but barring complications, it is likely that the source of your lower back discomfort is a form of overuse. Always remember that our bodies thrive with a diversity of movement and frequently alternating periods of rest and activity.

Understand your pelvic movements to be the core variable determining the health of your whole midsection as a hairstylist. Leading a movement with the pelvis will spare the upper back, arms and neck from strain. Furthermore the tilt of the pelvis controls the position (and therefore the state) of the lower back. If I could train a hairstylist's movement patterns from scratch, I would focus heavily on training healthy use of the pelvis.

Use the pelvis like it was a rolling pin. Even a small amount of pelvic tilt creates a significant change in the position of the lower back. Tilting the pelvis forward increases the curve in your lower back and tilting it backwards decreases it. It is also a good idea to stand with one leg resting on an object from time to time. This allows you to maintain healthy pelvic and spinal posture while resting the hard-working gluteal muscles one side at a time. When you engage your pelvic and leg muscles, the muscles in your upper back and neck and arms do not have to work as hard. The leg muscles are the biggest and strongest muscles in the body. When using them well, you might start feeling the 'post-workout' soreness rather than the nagging painful aches typical after a long day.

WRIST

In order to be healthy and effective the wrist needs to spend most of its time in a neutral position. When the wrist is flexed all the way down or extended all the way up, the nerves and blood vessels within are compressed. Repetitive movements outside a safe range of movement will take a significant toll on the wrist over time.

If you have pain in the wrist and a tender muscles in the forearm, then it would be important for you to re-calibrate the movements of your wrists and fingers.

Be mindful of the particular movements you make throughout the day and what proportion of them take the wrist beyond a reasonably neutral position. Ensure that your wrists do not tilt much to the left or right as you use scissors, combs and dryers. Use the elbow, shoulder and even pelvis to re-arrange your body position to reduce the need for extreme bending of the wrist. Techniques to resolve pain in the wrist and tension in the forearm muscles are offered in the chapter on Pain & How to Fix it.

NECK

The neck is strained when it drifts too far forward or is held in an asymmetrical position for too long. Keep your chin gently tucked and let your head rest directly on top of your neck.

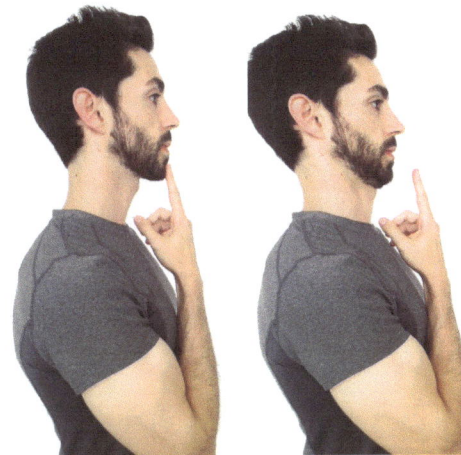

Correcting neck posture

The appropriate amount to tuck your chin can be tested by placing your index finger on your chin and then without moving your finger, head or neck, move your chin away from your finger. You should create about an inch of space.

Be patient with yourself and just keep reminding yourself to bring your head back to neutral when you catch it drifting forward or tilting too often. It will soon become habit. Mastering good shoulder blade posture will also contribute to better neck posture.

To recap, an ideal working posture entails a tucked chin, relaxed neck, shoulder blades pulled down and together, the pelvis tilted forward, gluteal muscles activated, and knees slightly bent. Ideal working behavior entails frequent changes in posture and type of movement.

Ergonomic Use of Equipment

BARBER CHAIR

The primary decisions guiding your use of the chair are dictated by your technical needs and working methods, as they should be. However, much of the way you use your chair can be improved to decrease the strain on your arms, shoulders, neck and low back.

One of the main challenges I witness stylists

struggle with is that a low chair means straining your low back and a high chair means straining your shoulders and upper back.

Adjusting the height of the chair to suit an optimal postural position for each task being performed is ideal. Otherwise, generally, the lower the chair the better *if* you are using your legs to keep you low and not your low back. When in one position for a while, you can help yourself reduce strain by rotating through these 4 stances.

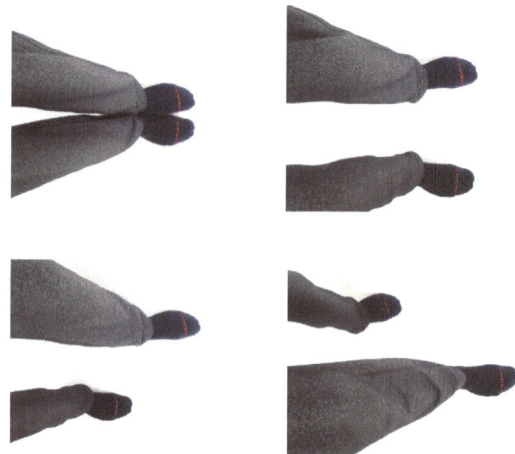

Using your legs more will initially be difficult and will leave you with tired legs at first. The alternative is moving more from you low back, which will lead to pain and problems. While working on using your legs more, you may be tempted to slip back into lazy habits. Fight the urge and remind yourself that by working on good posture you are getting stronger and living longer!

If you have the tendency to lift a chair really high, you are likely working with shoulders above 90 degrees, which is extremely tough on the joint and will wear your shoulders out prematurely. Train yourself to always keep the shoulders in proper posture (with shoulder blades together and down) and keep the elbow below the shoulder. You will have to compensate by moving your feet more and by adjusting the height of the chair more frequently, but if you value having working shoulders, you can justify working to develop this habit.

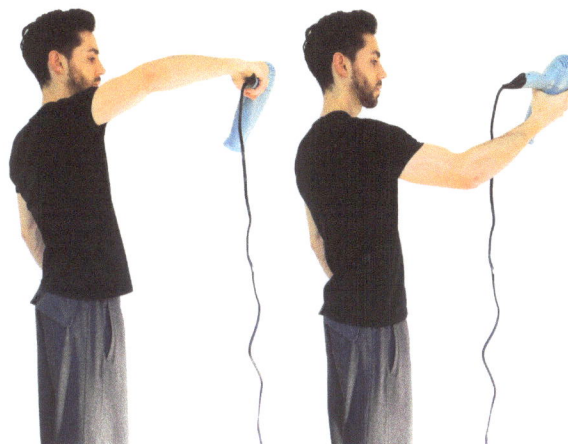

BAD   **GOOD**

BLOW DRYER

The most important thing to do when using a blow dryer is minimize movement of the wrist. This is accomplished by holding the dryer by its body, holding it closer to your body, creating movement more with fingers and with the elbow. Although many stylists are taught to hold the dryer by the handle, there are more drawbacks than advantages to holding it by the handle. It increases the strain on your already-overworked shoulders and wrists significantly. Holding the body of the dryer keeps your shoulder below 90°, sparing you a

significant amount of strain in your neck, upper back and shoulder muscles. It requires less movement in the wrist to shift the aim of the dryer and also spares the forearm muscles the strain of gripping a smaller handle.

When practicing holding the dryer by the body, you may need to lower the chair and increase how much you move around the client with your legs (thereby decreasing the amount of arm reaching required).

When you reduce excess movement at the wrist and keep the shoulder below 90° with more effective use of the chair, you will be able to work more proficiently and avoid developing painful problems.

If you don't like to hold the dryer by the body yet, invest in developing the habit. It makes a big difference. You will benefit from the increased efficiency of the arm movement, your shoulder and forearm muscles will last longer before getting tired and sore, and most importantly you will avoid wearing down your joints. It is also good to note that the cord from the dryer should be hanging down on the inside of your arm (closer to your body). This is important because when the cord is hanging outside your arm it pulls your wrist into external rotation and can cause a lot of specific repetitive strain.

SHEARS

Your hands naturally use standard shears relatively efficiently and finger problems are not all that common among stylists. It's important to find the style of shears best suited for you, to optimize wrist posture when cutting, and learn to stretch the thumb and forearm muscles regularly (since they are the most prone to muscle strain from scissor use). Also important is the use of good hygienic first aid practices when you cut the skin on your hand (yes, even tiny little cuts).

Like anything we do excessively however, we are prone to straining specific tissues. For those who do experience pain or problems when using scissors, it is important to test various styles of scissors (balanced, blade-heavy, off-set, semi-offset, swivel, crane, etc.) before committing to one kind. The small muscles and tendons of your hands and fingers will work slightly differently with each different type of scissor. The most ergonomic type of scissor is therefore the scissor you like best. No set of shears work perfectly for everyone, so shop around and test different styles. Spend at least two weeks with new shears before you commit to them. If your hands get sore or if you experience pain in your thumb or fingers when you work, it is a good indication that the scissors you use are not right for you. Pay close attention to finger/hand discomfort.

Beyond just hand and finger movement, it is valuable to consider how the way you use shears effects the rest of your body. Recent innovations in the design of ergonomic shears can help to significantly reduce the strain on your wrist, elbow, shoulder, neck and even your back. With Exthand shears for instance, your palm faces up while cutting, preventing the need to elevate the shoulder and elbow.

The cost of working with shears not well suited for you is far greater than the initial investment of a quality set. Always make sure the blades are sharp (sharpen at least every 8 months) and ensure the tension screws are not over-tightened.

SPIN BRUSH

Use the spin brush with a relaxed hand, wrist in neutral and use the tips of your fingers to rotate it. If you have pain in your fingers, hands, wrists or forearms, be careful not to underestimate the significance of your gripping technique. Every small change, every small improvement you can make helps you become more efficient and prevents injury in the future. Keeping your wrist in healthy positions is incredibly important, and most stylists do not have good form naturally.

Our bodies are very smart and we move in ways that accomplish our desired task most efficiently (but not necessarily the most safe).

Practice and remember that small changes make a big difference. Many stylists strain muscles and develop tennis elbow from gripping the spin brush with the whole hand. When gripping firmly, you are using the wrist to rotate it, pulling the wrist up and back excessively and moving the fingers too much.

Try to relax all the forearm muscles as best you can. Avoid a full hand grip of the brush (which causes too much wrist rotation). Use your fingers more. It is very important that you prevent tilting the wrist too much to either side; as shown in the image to the right.

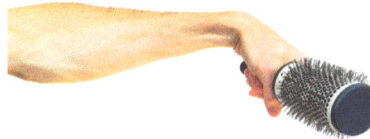
BAD

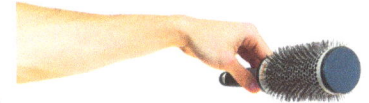
GOOD

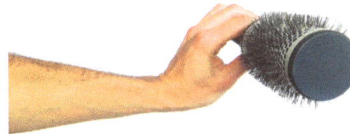
BAD

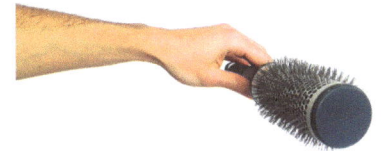
GOOD

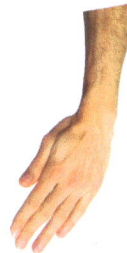
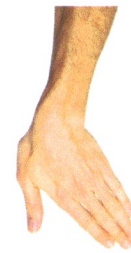

STOOL

Using a stool sporadically is a great way to keep your body happy. It interrupts the cycle of repetitive strain on the tissues of your low back and legs. Using a stool is sometimes convenient and sometimes inconvenient; which is perfect! Sitting some of the time and standing some of the time is the best way to ensure neither position strains your body too much. Using a height-adjustable saddle stool with wheels makes it easy to pop up and down. A saddle-shaped seat encourages a good neutral spine posture. I highly recommend using a stool occasionally, especially for those with back pain.

SINK/WASHING STATION

A common source of low back strain among salon workers, washing and rinsing clients at the sink is hard on the body because of having to bend forward for prolonged periods of time. The good news is that it can be done in a way that strengthens your body and prevents low back pain. The bad news is that it's not easy.

There is an exercise many people do in the gym called a deadlift. It's basically bending forward to pick up a weighted barbell off the ground. It's a great example of how something can be very good for your body or very damaging depending on how you do it. With good form, deadlifts are a great way to develop the strength of the gluteals and back muscles. If done improperly, the spine can suffer a lot of strain.

The same idea applies to activities like washing hair at the salon. The time you spend bent over the sink can contribute to strengthening your body or damaging your low back, depending on how you do it. That's an important idea, let that sink in for a minute. It's only different from doing deadlifts in the gym in that you are holding a position for prolonged periods of time rather than moving up and down.

While trying to improve your posture at the sink, be patient, it isn't easy and it takes time to feel the progress you are making. Optimize your bent over posture by doing the following; Start with your feet shoulder width apart. Bend your knees slightly. 'Spread the floor' – push lightly outwards with your feet. Curve your low back and stick your bum out a little. Keep your spine straight and shoulders together. Bend up and down at the hips, not the low back. Allow yourself to shift often and take frequent micro-breaks from your new (better, but more energy consuming) posture.

- - - - - - - - - - - - - - - - -

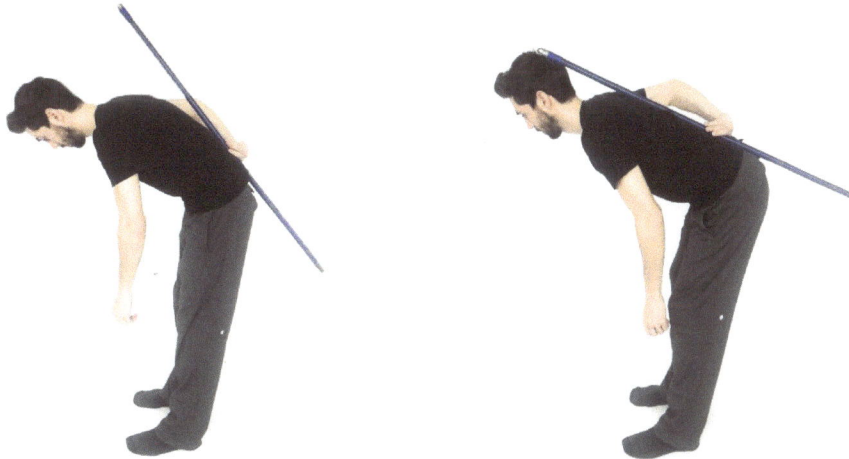

Test your bending form with a broomstick. Bend at the hips and keep your spine aligned with the stick.

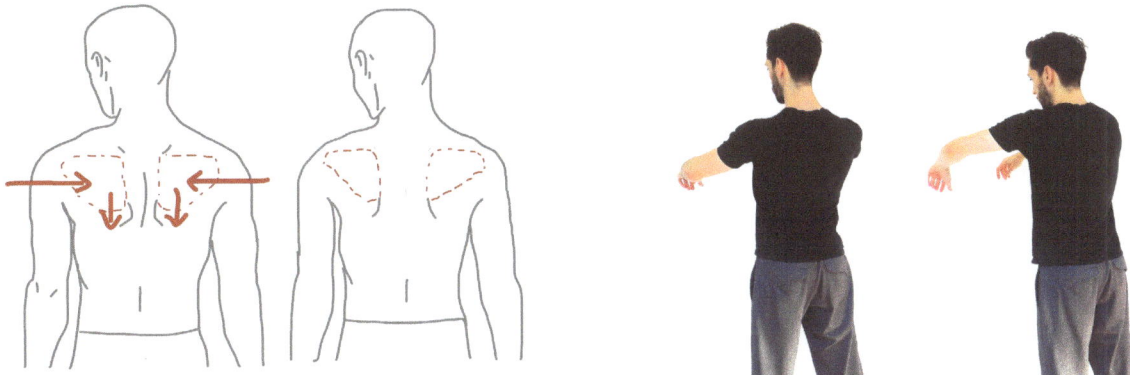

Remind yourself to keep your shoulder blades pulled back and down while you are reaching your arms forward.

4

Choosing Good Footwear

'Give a girl the right shoes, and she can conquer the world.'
– Marilyn Monroe

CHOOSING GOOD FOOTWEAR

Under the right conditions your feet are very happy to be used all day every day. They are designed to absorb forces and they do so very effectively. We only develop foot problems when there is an imbalance or excess. Excluding excess weight or a short leg (more common than most people think!), our feet tend only to become problematic when they are not supported adequately or are cramped in poorly fitting shoes constantly. Like all of the other areas of our bodies, the tissues of our feet also need variety.

Shoes without lateral support, arch support or heel support are not doing their job to support your feet. Considering how much time you spend standing and walking, it is well worthwhile to invest in finding suitable footwear.

TYPES OF SHOES

Choosing a good shoe has little to do with the type or brand. Even among a single line of a single brand, each shoe is unique, which is why it is valuable to know how to assess them. These days shoe design is predominantly shaped by fashion, leaving ergonomic value to be a secondary or tertiary consideration. If we follow a few simple rules however, it isn't difficult to find shoes you like that also offer the support you need.

Support can be taken to mean both the stiffness of the sole as well as how well it matches the contours of your foot. It is important because the bottoms of your feet are full of sensors that are constantly assessing the amount of pressure going through the specific areas of your feet. Your feet use this sensory input to coordinate the right sequences of muscle activation to move your feet and legs efficiently. This means that the quality of movement in your feet and ankles depends on having good support.

The feet and ankles are comprised of dozens of complex joints and are constantly performing intricately coordinated movements. When we wear footwear with soft, floppy, or poorly designed soles, we are diluting the ability of our feet to send these signals measuring pressure as they sense it. Good support therefore entails a hard sole that has contours that match our feet and that bend in the way our feet bend. Using the three tests described on page 36 is the best way to determine whether a sole is sufficiently stiff. If a shoe is comfortable, without pressure points and doesn't lead to soreness after several hours of wearing them, we can assume the contours of the sole and insole are adequately matched to your foot.

Finding the perfect amount of cushioning is sometimes a process of trial and error, but there are some shortcuts. Do not just go out looking for the softest insoles you can find. Too much cushion will degrade the biomechanical functioning of your feet and ankles. At the same time too little cushioning is not good either, a lack of cushioning will quickly lead to sore and strained feet. Cushioning in general decreases the rate of your foot's deceleration upon ground contact, thereby protecting your bones and joints. It's a matter of finding the right amount of cushion to reduce the impact of forces going through your feet while still allowing for firm ground contact. Experimenting with different insoles is a good idea. Give each attempt at least a week before deciding to stick with them. When shopping for insoles, a quick test of the height of your arches is helpful.

If you are able to stick three fingers under the arch of your foot while standing, burying the fingertips past the first phalange (tiny finger bone), then you should start with thicker cushioning. When upgrading the insoles that come with your shoes with cushioned 'aftermarket' insoles, don't forget to take the original ones out.

If you are only able to get one or two fingers under the arch of your foot, and not all the way past the

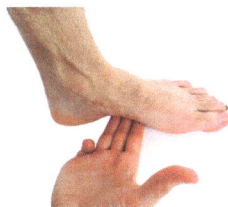

first phalanges, then you should be looking for more support and using less cushioning. Consider either custom orthotics or thin, simple store bought insoles.

When shopping for shoes, I recommend being weary of shoe salespeople who discuss anatomy or biomechanics. Considering the complexity of your body, it would be much wiser to stick to the principles laid out in this section when deciding on a shoe, or to consult a specialist. I often hear of people being sold shoes because they are 'made for people with flat feet' or 'made for pronators'. This is an oversimplification and can lead to more harm than good. Seek such advice from a healthcare professional.

Orthotics are valuable, but only for some people. My recommendation is to first use store bought insoles with good shoes. If you continue to experience chronic foot problems, *then* consider being assessed for orthotics. Podiatrists, pedorthists, chiropractors and a few other types of practitioners can make custom orthotics.

There are three quick and easy tests to perform on any shoe to determine quality and biomechanical sufficiency. They are demonstrated on the next page.

- - - - - - - - - - - - - - - - -

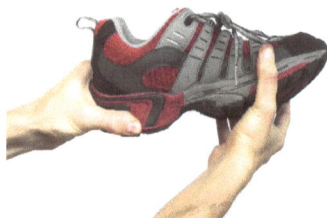 **Pass**

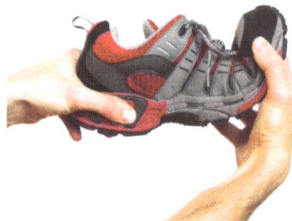 **Pass**

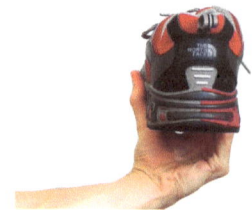 **Pass**

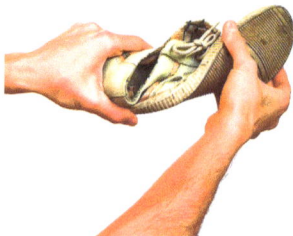 **Fail**

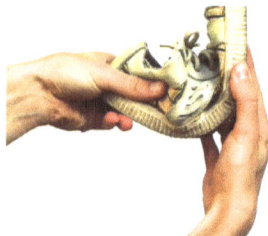 **Fail**

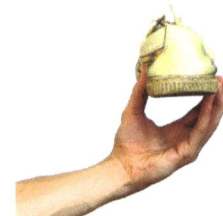 **Fail**

Twist test

First, hold the heel and front of the shoe and twist in different directions. The sole of a shoe should NOT easily give when twisted like a rag. It passes the test if it is very stiff and does not collapse easily. This tests the lateral support of a shoe.

Toe bend test

For a shoe to be biomechanically suitable it must bend at a point just behind the metatarsal heads to an angle of about 30 degrees. When bending the sole back on itself, the bend of the sole should occur ONLY where the ball of your foot goes and NOT in the middle.

Straight heel test

Place the shoe on a flat surface and look at the heel of the shoe, make sure it is straight upright and perpendicular to the surface it lies on. This seems like a silly thing to check, but the reality is that a great number of shoes end up with crooked heels as the result of sloppy manufacturing. A crooked heel will not only be uncomfortable, but will fail to provide the posterior support you need.

HEELS

Wearing high heels can be tough on your body- if done sloppily. However, if done properly, it can be well-tolerated. First we will learn the effect wearing heels has on your anatomy, and then explore techniques that mitigate the damage from wearing them frequently.

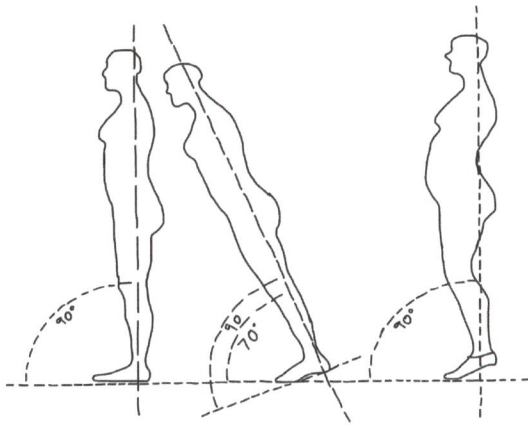

Wearing heels shortens the calf muscles, puts extra pressure on the ball of your foot, compresses your toes together, strains the hamstrings and increases the pressure on your low back. If not worn responsibly, they can lead to hammer-toe, bunions, permanent muscle shortening, tendonitis, changes in spinal posture, and can even contribute to the deterioration of the vertebral discs in your low back.

But there's an upside! Wearing heels can help develop your ankle balance (assuming you don't sprain them in the process), can challenge you to improve your upper back and neck posture, can shift the pressure points on your knees, shift the strain through muscles in your low back and of course help you look sexy.

Be smart about it, and you can minimize the damage and maximize the gains. Here are a few tips;

Vary the height - even if you have a favorite pair of pumps, switch it up. If you are wearing heels all day or for consecutive days, wear heels of different height. The more of a difference there is the better. It changes the strain on your feet and body and will decrease the chance of injuring tissues.

Carry sneaky purse flats - many a smart lady I know sneaks a pair of flats or ballet slippers into her purse when leaving home with heels. This is smart because there is always a good chance you will be going for a long impromptu stroll at some point, or have some time alone when you can give your body a rest. The bigger the heels, the more grateful your feet will be to have slippers.

Stretch! Your calves take the biggest beating, being shortened right up and still having to work hard. Start with the calves (G-1), and then stretch the hamstrings (F-1) and the low back (E-1). You can even roll your foot over top a ball (G-2) or bottle to offer your plantar fascia some relief.

Consider custom orthotics - A few orthotic manufacturers make special orthotics for high heels. Keep in mind however that regular shaped orthotics (that look like a typical shoe insole) are *not* the same thing. Good high heel orthotics will have a hook shape for the heel and a thick middle section.

The orthotic will help by redistributing the forces that travel through the ball of your foot. This will increase comfort and can reduce the likelihood of developing painful bunions. One challenge you may face with these is that they can sometimes take up too much space in the heel, making for a difficult fit in some shoes. Remember to bring them with you when buying new shoes.

Using these few tips regularly will help offset the strain that wearing heels puts on your body. But that doesn't mean you can forget to exercise moderation. Switch it up, stretch it out, sneak those flats and see your podiatrist, then go ahead and wear your heels guilt (and pain) free!

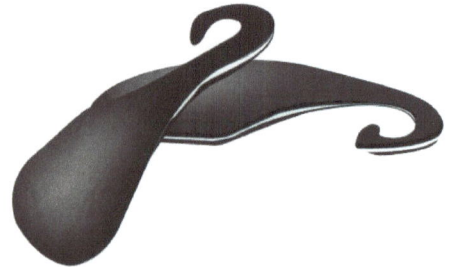

STRETCHES TO COUNTER THE EFFECTS OF WEARING HEELS

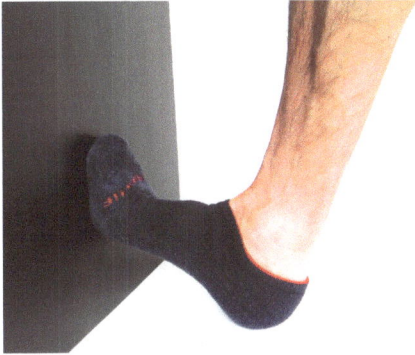

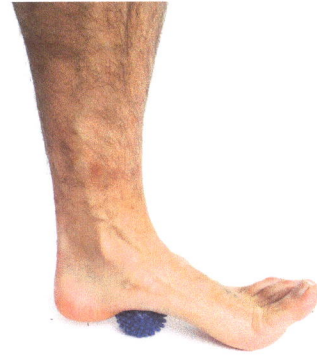

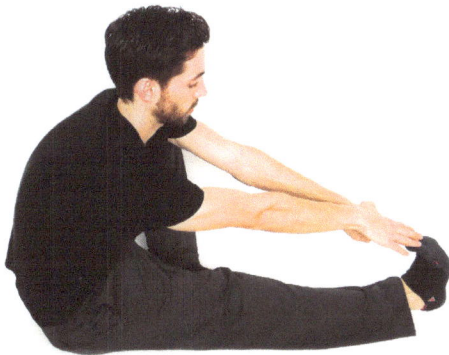

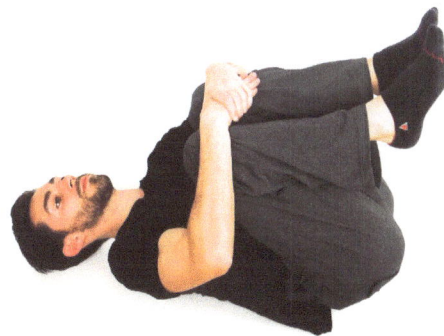

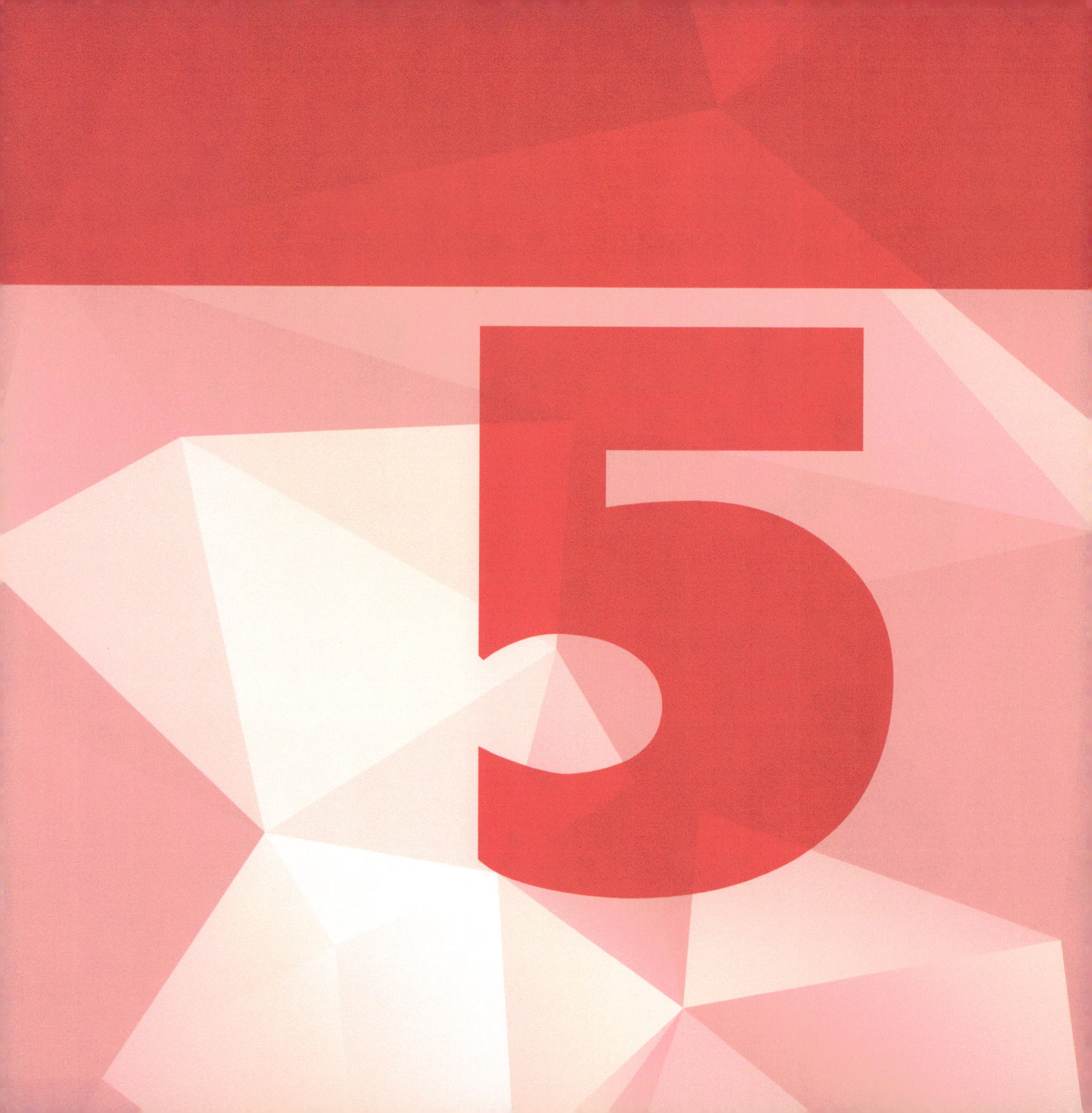

5

Common Mistakes

"We cannot change anything unless we accept it."

- Carl Jung

COMMON MISTAKES

It is helpful to understand that our bodies are designed to work very efficiently, and that in certain circumstances this can work against us. We instinctively move our bodies in ways that will accomplish a task in the quickest possible way, but not necessarily the safest. When we perform a task such as blow drying repetitively for hours a day all the time, the strain can become too much for our hand, wrist and forearm. It is immensely valuable to take the chance to assess the quality of our most common movements and modify the way we do certain things to accommodate the volume at which we do them.

Reaching forward repetitively will compromise the integrity of your shoulder joint and adds extra strain on the muscles that move your arm. This is the most common cause for shoulder pain among hairstylists. Reaching is necessary of course, but the position of your shoulder blades makes a substantial difference in how the time you spend reaching forward effects you. Training yourself to keep your shoulder blades down and back will ensure that your shoulders are happy by keeping the joint in a more neutral position and by drawing the larger stronger muscles into your work, sparing the smaller more susceptible ones.

Begin with exercises B 1, 2 & 3 to start training that healthy shoulder blade position. Continue into more advanced exercises found in the next chapter if needed. Keeping your shoulder blades down and back also has a significant impact on neck posture, helping to keep the head back in a neutral position.

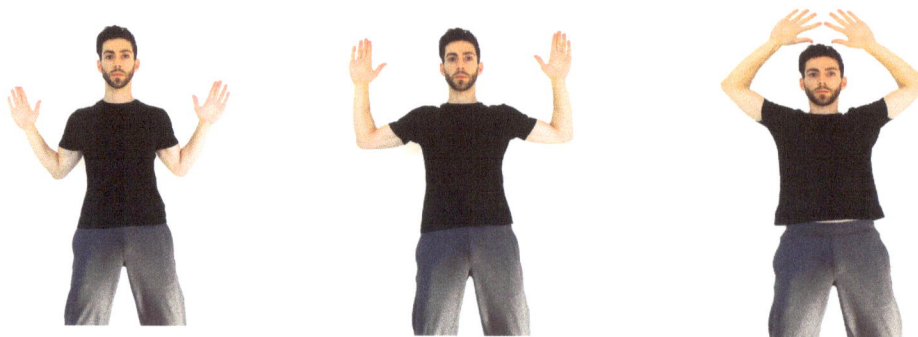

B 1. Wall angels. Stand with all of your back against a wall, feet a foot from the wall and knees slightly bent. Slowly move your arms up and down 10 times, keeping wrists AND elbows against the wall the entire time.

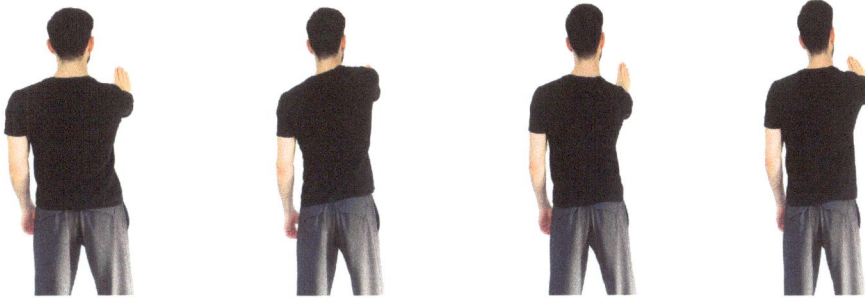

B 2. Wall clocks. Stand facing a wall, placing your palm against the wall with your arm straight. Without moving your hand, move your shoulder clockwise from the 12 o'clock position then to 3 to 6 & to 9. Move slowly and keep everything still except the shoulder.

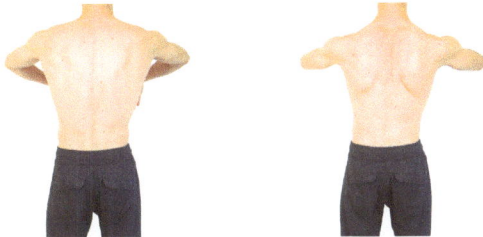

B 3. Shoulder blade in the back pocket. Squeeze your shoulder blades together and then downwards without moving your arms. Practice holding them in that position while moving your arms.

Working with your elbows higher than your shoulders should be avoided as much as possible. Lowering the client's chair and modifying the way you hold a dryer or brush are the easiest and best ways to reduce the time your arms spend way up there in the danger zone. The position your arms are in when holding your elbow up at shoulder height is detrimental as it compresses the tendons of the rotator cuff muscles, potentially leading to tearing and tendonitis.

Twisting the wrist too often is the immediate cause of many common problems I see among hairstylists. Blow drying, using a spin brush and cutting all require significant movement at the wrist. If you suffer from wrist or hand pain, it will be valuable to re-organize movement habits of the wrists and arms. Among the most strenuous movements is holding the wrist outwards in the direction of the pinky finger, and holding the wrist up.

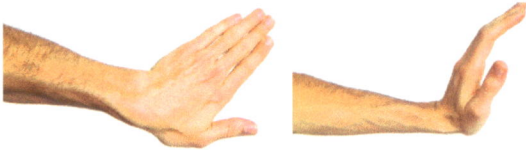

Correcting form of the wrist is one of the more difficult habits to re-train. It takes discipline and practice.

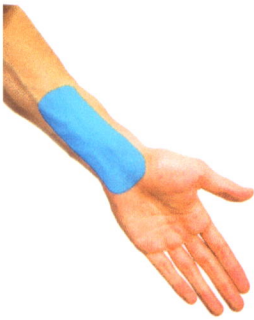

To reduce the amount of wrist bending or twisting required with any activity, we need to learn to use more of the rest of our arms and shoulders. One helpful way to help re-train wrist movements is using kinesiology tape, which increases your sensitivity to damaging wrist movements.

Shifting the head too far forward is a form of body language that demonstrates an increase in focus. We move our eyes closer to the object of our focus, tilt our head and extend it forward to demonstrate that we are paying close attention. But it doesn't actually help us do a better job. In fact, the more controlled and laid back we appear, the more we seem like an expert.

Recall the optimal position of the shoulder blades and always remind yourself to keep your chin slightly tucked. This will ensure your neck posture remains optimal and will reduce the tension being put on the muscles at the back of your head and neck. This will in turn reduce the pain in your neck and reduce the chances of developing tension headaches.

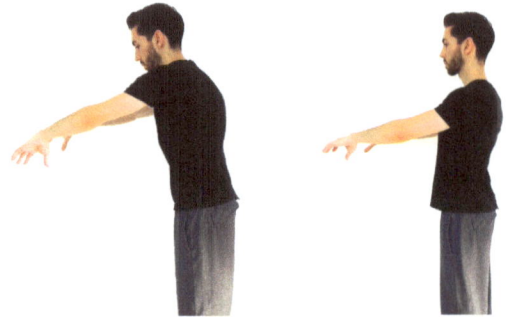

The second position demonstrates the optimal position of shoulders and neck

Having feet too close together has no practical benefit, but we do it because it allows us to turn off pelvic muscles and saves energy. Your work requires you to be constantly moving side to side, so keeping your feet together will lead to a lot of extra strain throughout your torso. Keeping your feet at least a foot apart from one another will increase the activation of the muscles in your thigh and pelvis - the strongest muscles of your body.

Leaning on one hip too often is a habit very easy to get into. It's alright to do occasionally while leaning up against a wall waiting for a bus, but tilting your pelvis to one side while you work throws your whole body off and puts extra strain on that hip joint. The effects of spending time leaning on one hip span from head to toe. We are most inclined to hip lean when our gluteus medius muscles are tired or weak. These muscles are very important in our standing posture, walking and running technique. A large number of people I come across in practice have significantly weak gluteus medius muscles. This is because people generally sit too much (keeping the muscles inactive) and don't do much that challenge this set of muscles.

If you are a chronic hip leaner, a good first step is to shift over to the other hip every time your catch yourself doing it. This will increase your awareness of it. The next step is to use your bum. As silly as it sounds, squeezing your cheeks together will activate your gluteal muscles and make you feel more squarely grounded. The third step is to start doing a side-lying gluteus medius leg raise exercise (F- 2). Alternatively you could take up a racquet sport or start doing crab walks (F-3).

Wearing poor footwear is a serious mistake. With unsupportive footwear your whole body suffers, not just your feet. The people making and selling shoes don't prioritize the effect their shoe has on your skeletal alignment. You you need to make sure that your shoe does more for you than look nice. Refer to the chapter on Choosing Good Footwear to learn how to test a shoe before you buy it.

- - - - - - - - - - - - - - - - -

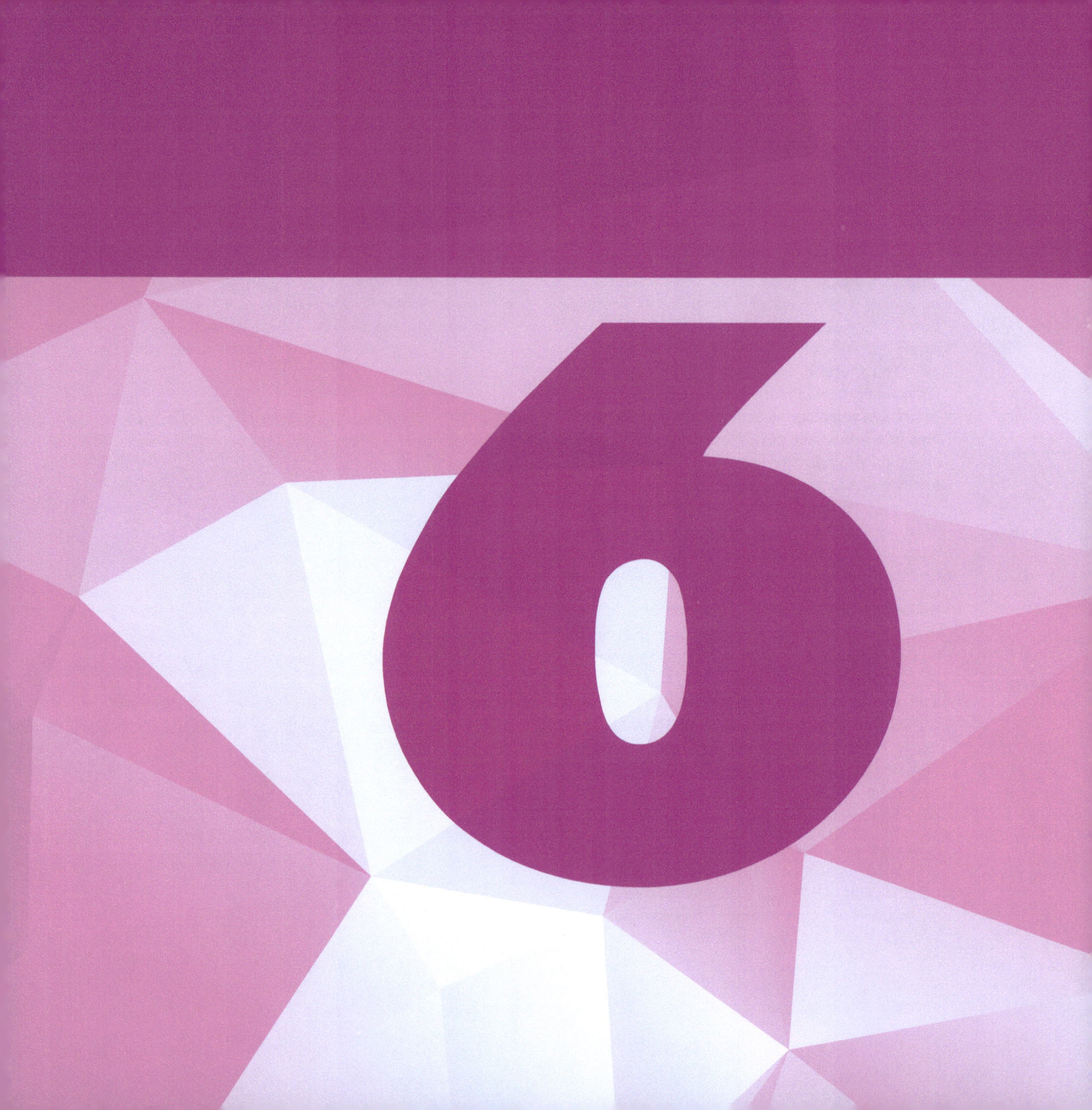

6

Pain And How To Fix It

"If you desire healing, let yourself fall ill."

- Rumi

PAIN AND HOW TO FIX IT

The most important part of dealing with pain is figuring out precisely what the problem is. This section is intended to be a rough guide to managing simple regional pains. It is still wise to consult the next section on specific injuries and conditions and to seek a clinical diagnosis from your doctor.

If your pain is new and mild, you can begin by treating yourself, then work to identify and address the cause of your pain. If your problem persists beyond a few weeks, is severe or interferes with your regular activities, then it is wise to promptly seek appropriate help. Treating yourself can entail resting, stretching, massaging, using topical therapies, ice, over-the-counter pain killers, taping, and other remedies. Identifying the cause is a matter of listening to your body and paying attention to the activities that aggravate the pain. You can use the insight you gain to modify your activities, then improve your habits and your movements.

Keep in mind, the tools I use and recommend have many alternatives. For instance, you can use a tennis ball or lacrosse ball instead of an Acuball for many of the applications. A golf ball can substitute for an acuball mini.

The symbols below represent the type of therapeutic options recommended

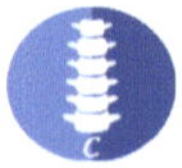

Chiropractic

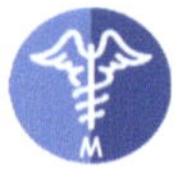

Medical

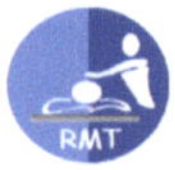

Massage (Registered Massage Therapist)

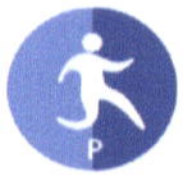

Physiotherapy

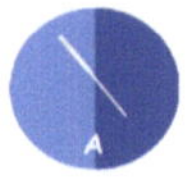

Acupuncture

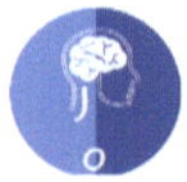

Osteopathy

Visual depictions of the body parts discussed throughout this chapter

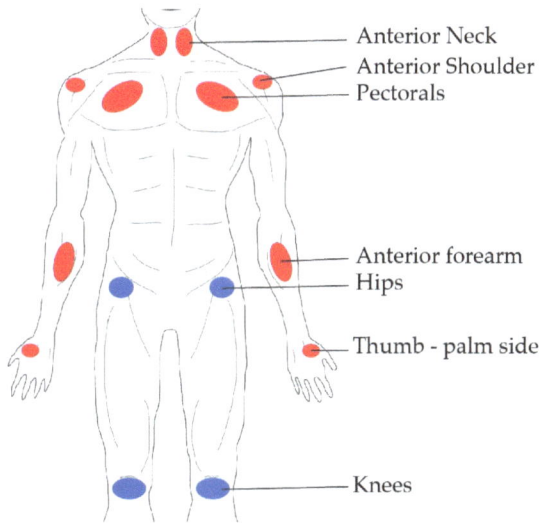

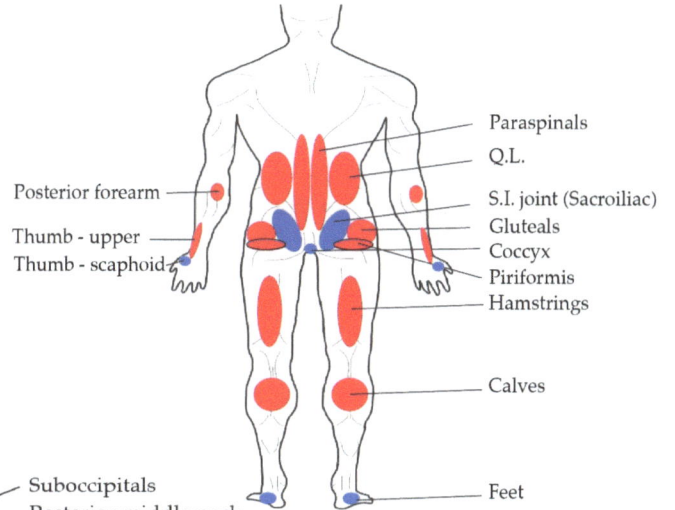

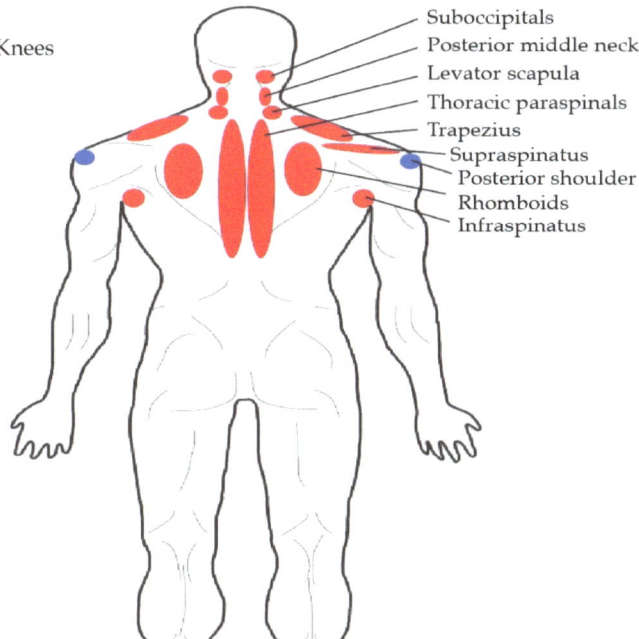

Anterior Neck
Anterior Shoulder
Pectorals

Anterior forearm
Hips

Thumb - palm side

Knees

Paraspinals
Q.L.
Posterior forearm
S.I. joint (Sacroiliac)
Gluteals
Thumb - upper
Coccyx
Thumb - scaphoid
Piriformis
Hamstrings

Calves

Feet

Suboccipitals
Posterior middle neck
Levator scapula
Thoracic paraspinals
Trapezius
Supraspinatus
Posterior shoulder
Rhomboids
Infraspinatus

Throughout the book, exercises and stretches are referred to with a corresponding code (e.g. A-1 or B-2). The code directs you to the exercise in the Exercise Appendix featured near the back of the book.

Thumb- Palm side - There are two small groups of muscles here that move the thumb called the flexor opponens and adductor opponens muscles. These muscles can become tight and painful with repetitive scissor use.

Your scissor thumb needs to be taken care of. It can handle a lot and it doesn't often act up even when used all day every day. So when it does, we need to deal with it promptly so it doesn't interfere with work. Firstly, if pain in the thumb is recurring, it is time to reconsider the shears you use. Next, take into account other activities or hobbies you have that may be contributing to the strain. It can be anything that requires prolonged use of the thumb to grip, pull or push. Modify the way you use the thumb or drop the activity temporarily until you recover. Once you are confident that you are using the scissors best fit for you (more in the chapter on Optimal Biomechanics) and that you don't have any unnecessary extraneous activities, then it's time to treat the muscles. To treat sore thumb muscles, find the most tender point in the area and apply a moderate amount of pressure with

your other thumb. Place your sore thumb on the edge of any surface and move your hand down to extend the thumb back, stretching the thumb muscles (C-2-3). Push firmly on the tender point for 15 seconds while holding the thumb in this position (C-1). Repeat three times. Do this twice a day for three days.

Use the acuball mini (take a look at the Helpful Tools section to see images of the acuball and other tools I refer to) to massage the group of tight thumb muscles. Follow this with pressing firmly on both sides of the thumb muscles for 30 seconds 3 times (C-50). Alternatively, roll tension out using C-49.

Mobilize the thumb and wrist to reduce tension in the joints with C-28 and C-48.

Help prevent further pain in the area by:

Tilting the wrist slightly towards the thumb while working to limit excessive thumb muscle activity.

Once the pain has been gone for a week or longer, begin playing with a stress ball for 10 minutes a day in both hands. It's easy when you make it a habit during idle time - in between clients, watching T.V., walking, talking on the phone or even reading.

Thumb - scaphoid area

*If you have recently fallen on your hand or wrist and have pain in this area, you may have a fractured scaphoid bone and should see your doctor.

Pain in this area is typically the result of extending the thumb back too much, using scissors that have too much resistance or tilting the wrist towards the pinky finger too often while working. Begin by doing 8 gentle repetitions of the C-28 wrist mobilization twice each day.

Minimize the strain on the thumb and wrist by ensuring your scissors are sharp (sharpen at least every eight or nine months). Also make sure to not over-tighten tension screws. Use balanced scissors, a blade-heavy pair will increase the strain on your thumb and wrist. Play around with different styles, although offset or swivel scissors are often comfortable, there isn't any one type of scissor that works perfectly for everyone.

Once the pain has subsided, begin doing 30 slow repetitions of the elastic band stretch three times each week (C-4). Stop if the exercise begins to aggravate the area.

Thumb - upper area

A commonly problematic area for hairstylists, pain in this area is typically the result of an inflamed tendon from excessive wrist movements. Specifically, bending the thumb and wrist together towards the pinky finger too often will aggravate the tissues along the thumb side of the wrist and forearm.

Remember to keep the wrist out of this position.

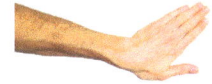

Use a piece of kinesiology tape on the thumb side of your wrist. Apply it with some tension with your wrist in a neutral position. Alternatively put one ring of kinesiology tape around the wrist where it becomes the hand and another one inch further up.

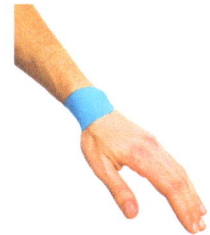

Symptoms can be improved by massaging the forearm.

Press firmly on the muscle belly near the elbow (of extensor carpi radialis) until you find a tender point. Continue to apply firm pressure on the tender point while you stretch the wrist down (C-5). Perform the same maneuver on the muscle called brachioradialis (C-51).

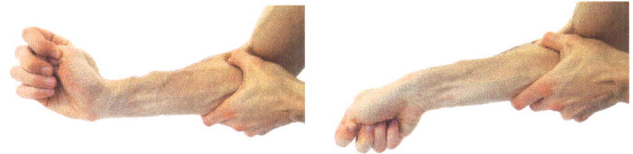

Minimize activities or wrist movements which aggravate the area.

Once the pain has subsided, begin to strengthen your forearm muscles using the Theraband Flexbar

(C-6). Progressively increase the frequency during the first week, but stop if the pain returns.

Begin with both wrists up (as if you were riding a motorcycle), start by twisting down with only the good hand, then slowly (the slower the better) allow the injured arm to let the tension down until the bar is back in neutral. Begin again by bringing the bar back up with both wrists (C-6).

Alternatively we can use a resistance band attached to either a solid object or your foot, begin with the wrist bent back and lift the arm until the band is tight (C-7). Then slowly let your wrist bend down without moving the rest of your arm. Perform 3 sets of 10 reps for 3 weeks. Here we are strengthening the forearm muscles in a specific way that will lead to better movement and less injury.

Once you have resolved the pain, the key to keeping it away will be training yourself to keep your wrist out of the 'bad' position when working (refer to section on optimal biomechanics).

Posterior Middle Neck

The most common causes of serious neck pain are muscle strains, whiplash, disc herniations, and facet irritation. If your neck pain developed very quickly and is significant, it may be one of the above. In that case you can read about each of these conditions on your way to the doctors office. If you're pain has come on progressively over time and is proportional to the

amount of time you spend working, then you likely have a postural strain. You may be straining your neck muscles by either constantly bending your neck down or by letting your head drift forward. Remember to tuck your chin in slightly (midway between normal and double chin). Keeping your shoulder blades together and down will also ensure better neck posture.

In the short term, you can find relief from targeted stretching techniques (A-8,9 and B-11) and from using an acuball (A-1-2-3).

Next, try the towel cradle mobilization by lying on your back with a rolled up towel cradling the back of your head. Try to relax your neck as much as possible while you slowly rock your head from side to side with the 'handles' of the towel (A-4).

Note that sleeping on your stomach can contribute to tension and pain in this part of your neck. If you sleep on your stomach and are always feeling tight and sore through your neck, tape a tennis or squash ball onto the middle of your chest when you go to sleep each night. You can also just drop a ball into the front pocket of a T-shirt that you wear to sleep. Try that for a week and you may be surprised at how much of a difference it makes.

If your pain is chronic, or if you are over 50 years old, we must consider a degenerative condition like arthritis. It would be wise to visit your doctor and have X-rays taken to determine if this may be the case in your situation. But regardless of what your particular issue may be, strengthening the neck muscles will improve the condition of your neck in the long term. Rehabilitating the neck muscles is worthwhile because the payoff is great in both the short and long term. Life is a lot better when you can look over your shoulder without pain. The A-5 and A-6 exercises will facilitate better posture and more support for the vertebrae in your neck, reduce pain, reduce chances of future pain and even decrease headache frequency.

Using Kinesiology tape: place two strips along the back of the neck down to the mid-back while holding the neck in neutral and keeping the chin tucked. Apply moderate tension to the tape when applying. Use this application for a minimum of two weeks (each application should stay on for 4-5 days).

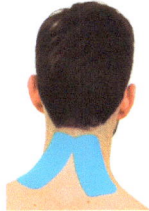

Suboccipitals

Tight suboccipital muscles can often contribute to tension headaches. These small muscles help to tilt the head up and rotate it. Pain on just one side is typically the result of a habit of rotating the head to one side more than the other. Release the tension by stretching with an acuball (A-7) or two golf balls side by side in a bag. 15 minutes on a heated acuball will significantly reduce the tension in these muscles (A-2).

Alternatively, try the standing stretch. Tuck your chin, bend your neck down, rotate slightly and pull your head down with your arm (A-8).

To prevent these muscles from getting tight and tender, we must develop the strength of the larger postural muscles in the neck.

Performing this one exercise on a regular basis will do the trick (A-5). The improvements you make when doing this exercise will also carry over to improve the condition of your upper back and neck in several other ways.

Lying on your back, tuck your chin all the way, lift your head off the ground about an inch and hold it there. Use a timer to test how long you can hold your head there without un-tucking your chin or shaking. Once you have a baseline time, do 8 repetitions of that time each day and monitor your times as they begin to improve. You should aim to hold for 35 seconds without losing form or shaking.

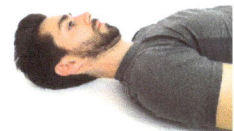

Trapezius

These muscles hold your shoulders up, and work extra hard when you keep them hunched up. It's rare for me to meet a hairstylist who does not have tension and tenderness in their traps. We should be invested in the health of these muscles because they affect the head (they can contribute to headaches), the neck, the upper back and the shoulders to a significant extent. The best way to prevent the trapezius muscles from getting tense and painful is by keeping the shoulder blades down, back and relaxed while you work. It is easier said than done and takes some training.

Stretching the trapezius is best done by sitting on one hand - as much of your hand as possible - so that you are not able to lift that shoulder, and then using the other arm to gently tilt the head in the opposite direction (A-9). It is also possible to stretch out your traps really well by doing the same stretch and having a friend push down (firmly but carefully) near the outer edge of the muscle (where it is still soft) (A-10). Releasing the tension in the muscle can also be done alone with B-34.

Properly applied kinesiology tape can help re-train your shoulder posture quite significantly. Tension the tape to 60-70% when applying.

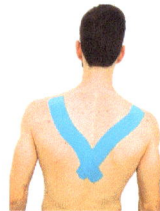

Posterior Forearm

Although it is common to have tight and painful muscles on the back of the forearm, it is often the result of holding your wrist up too frequently while you work. Remember to relax your wrist, keep it in neutral as much as possible, and use the rest of the body to help move the hand. Extensive blow-drying and use of the spin brush may aggravate these muscles. Review your form using the guidelines in the Optimal Biomechanics chapter.

To reduce tension in these muscles, stretch the muscles (C-10). Follow this by pushing a strait arm up against the wall with the back of your hand against the wall and fingers pointing down. With your other hand, push firmly on the tender areas and massage slowly with plenty of pressure (C-11). Using the acuball or flexbar on the muscles is helpful. If the focal point of the pain is right up by the elbow, consult the next section on tennis elbow.

Levator Scapula

Pain here? Not surprising. This little muscle goes from your shoulder blade to the vertebrae of your neck. It is involved in many movements, and is stretched out quite a bit when both your neck and arms are forward - as they are when you're working on hair. Even with good posture, it's hard to avoid overusing the levator scapula as a hairstylist. Treating the tension in these muscles can be a bit tricky so be patient. Here are the best options:

Have a friend use their thumb to push down very firmly half an inch above the most tender spot and hold the pressure there. Then you slowly bring your chin to your chest and rotate your head to the opposite direction, while keeping your shoulder down. Repeat 6 times (B-9). Treat yourself using an acuball mini or golf ball with tape around it (so it doesn't slip around). Lean up against a wall, place the ball on the tender area, push yourself into the ball, bring your head all the way

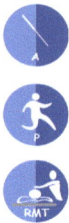

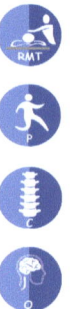

down and to the opposite shoulder, reach down to the floor with the arm of the same side, and then slowly start nodding your head. It's difficult so be patient and you will be glad you were (B-10). Alternatively you can use the acuball mini lying on your back. Roll around until you've found the tight tender spot, use your weight to let the ball press into the spot and then spent 5 minutes relaxing and breathing slowly.

For a quick stretch at work, sit down on your hand (with the palm up and right up to the wrist so that you can't raise your shoulder), use the opposite arm to pull your head all the way down and to the opposite direction. Hold this for 20 seconds and repeat twice (B-11).

Supraspinatus

The supraspinatus is in charge of lifting the arm up the first bit before the deltoids kick in. It is also one of the rotator cuff muscles, contributing significantly to intricate shoulder movements. We increase the load it bears when our shoulders are hunched, rolled forward or when our arms are turned inwards (as in a thumbs-down position).

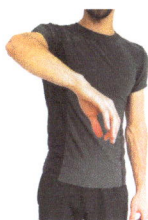

No wonder why they are so commonly strained!

Good upper body posture and movement habits are essential to keep the supraspinatus healthy. Review the Optimal Biomechanics section on shoulder posture. Simply put, the further your shoulder blades slide forward when you work, the more strain goes through your supraspinatus. Keeping your shoulder blades held back, together and down while you work will instantaneously reduce the workload of the supraspinatus.

If the pain has been present for more than 2 months, refer to the description of rotator cuff sprain in the conditions section and visit your doctor.

The best way to self-treat the supraspinatus is combining stretches and exercises.

Begin with exercises B-12, B-5, and B-13.

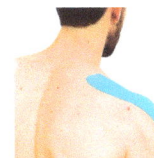

An application of kinesiology tape can be of short-term benefit.

Since the muscle is very superficial, using topical muscle relaxants can be effective. For long-term shoulder health, improve the strength of the muscle with the straight-arm thumbs up strengthening exercise (B-14). Use your choice of a resistance band or a small weight. The scapular clock exercise (B-2) improves the muscle coordination in the area, which will help you improve your shoulder posture and prevent unnecessary strain.

Posterior Shoulder Capsule

Sharp pains in the shoulder with certain movements is one of the cardinal signs of an irritated or injured capsule. The capsule is the sensitive casing around the glenohumeral joint. When irritated, it can hurt to move your arm into specific positions, hurt to sleep on the affected side and can refer pain down the front or side of the upper arm.

The first step in treating an upset capsule is with the pendulum exercise. On the affected side, hold anything that weighs a few pounds (dumbbell, can of soup, your cat), lean over and let your arm dangle. Start to slowly let your arm swing in small circles. Then focus on allowing all the muscles of your shoulder to relax, which will then stretch and loosen up the capsule (C-42).

Continue improving the capsule by stretching the pectorals for 6 minutes each day (B5 or B6), and doing 20 slow wall clocks each day (B2).

Try the table shoulder stretch (B-15). Lean forward overtop a waist-height table with your hands pointing in towards each other. Lean right down overtop of them with your elbows pointed out and then rotate slowly from side to side aiming to get your nose past each elbow.

Use the small acuball to release the tension of the muscles at the back of the arm - just above the armpit (B16).

Since most capsule issues of the shoulder are the result of an imbalance of the rotator cuff muscles, it is important to address weaknesses in your shoulder and arm working habits. If a capsule issue recurs, rehabilitative exercises should be done consistently for 3 months beyond the time when symptoms disappear.

Infraspinatus

This muscle rotates the arm outwards. It would be very active when reaching back for a seat belt in a car for example. It also works hard when the arm is reached forward with the elbow up and the wrist down. Because muscles are most taxed when both contracted and stretched simultaneously, holding a blow dryer up with a high elbow uses the infraspinatus quite intensely.

It is one of the rotator cuff muscles, which together are a bit like tent poles holding a tarp. When you are dealing with a rotator cuff muscle, you must make sure to deal with all of them together if you want to end up with happy shoulders.

The acuball can be used effectively to release tension in the rotator cuff muscles. Start with the ball between the spine and shoulder blade, then push up against a wall and slowly roll around while slowly moving your arm in various positions.

Stretch it gently by bending your elbow and then lifting your arm all the way up and using your other arm to stretch it further back (B-18). Stretching will help with the symptoms in the short term, strengthening will ensure your shoulder stays happy and healthy. Strengthening is best done with straight forward external rotation using a resistance band (B-19). This rehabilitative exercise should be accompanied by 3 sets of 10 wall angels (B-1) every day for 8 weeks. Stand with feet together and one foot away from the wall. Push as much of your back onto the wall as you can, including your head (but keeping your chin tucked is very important). Then, starting with the arms bent and parallel to the floor, and keeping both the elbows and wrists touching the wall, slowly (having slow and smooth movements is the key) move your arms up until the fingers touch. If your infraspinatus trouble persists, you'll need to spend time making improvements to your shoulder postural habits, particularly while at work.

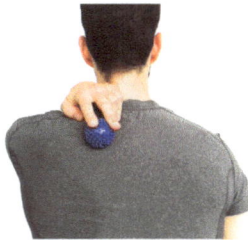

Rhomboids & Lower & Middle Traps

With such a heavy work load, it's no wonder that most people have sore, tight or problematic muscles here. The rhomboids and the lower traps are in charge of holding the shoulder blades in a retracted position (closer together). You use them A *lot*. These muscles operate most effectively when they are at normal length (as opposed to being stretched as the arms and shoulders reach forward). And like any other muscle, they need diversity of movement and resting breaks. This lends to the importance of working on good shoulder blade posture, strengthening the muscles outside of work, and stretching the muscles regularly while at work.

Stretching should be done twice daily. Use stretches B-20 & B-21.

The stretch for the pectoralis minor is important because you use these muscles a lot, and when they get tight they pull your shoulder forward, adding more strain to your back. Trunk rotation will gently work the muscles around your spine. Be careful not to do it too fast or too hard.

Mobilizing your shoulder blades is a good way to warm up and reset your shoulder and back muscles. Interlock your fingers 'inside out', keep your arms straight and slowly move your arms all the way forward and backwards without moving your torso as demonstrated in B-22 and B-23.

Child's Pose stretch is one of the best ways to get a good stretch in the lower mid back area (B-24).

A more advanced stretch is the swiss ball back stretch where you lie overtop a swiss ball with your mid back resting on it, stretch your arms up over your head and slowly let them fall back as far as they go (B-25). Hold the position for several seconds, return to the starting position and then repeat.

The sitting wall press (B-26) is a good way to release tension in your midback while strengthening the right muscles. Sit cross-legged with your back against a wall holding a bar or rod above your head. Slowly glide the bar up the wall and back down to your head while keeping as much of your body (focus on back, head and elbows) against the wall was possible.

Strengthening can also be done with a resistance band (B-27). Wrap the band around a secure object, grab both ends and pull the elbows back until the shoulder blades are pulled back and together all the way. Your arms should start straight and end bent.

The field goal exercise is a good alternative (B-28), where you lie on your stomach, 'put your shoulder blades in your back pocket' and hold that position while you raise your arms slowly into the 'field goal' position repeatedly.

The acuball mini is very useful to relax your rhomboids (B-29). Either lean up against a wall or lie on the floor, dig the ball in to the tight areas and move your arm slowly across your body.

Anterior Neck

Experiencing aches or pains in the front of the neck can be from tension in a muscle called the SCM (full name SternoCleidoMastoid) and is typically most tender near the bottom of the neck. If you are experiencing pain in the middle of the front of your neck, see your doctor.

SCM tenderness is most commonly caused by poor neck posture, whiplash injuries, and stomach sleeping. Improving the way you use your head and neck while you work is done predominantly by practicing to keep the chin tucked, the shoulder blades down and back, and keeping the head neutral on the neck.

Stretching the SCM (A-11) is very tricky, sometimes even dangerous and I generally recommend leaving it to a qualified therapist. A-12 demonstrates another advanced self- treatment protocol, which is quite effective - but should also be used with great caution. Do not proceed if it causes any pain in the back of the neck, light headedness or any other symptoms.

As it is with many other neck issues, the A-5 exercise is valuable here too. Lying on your back, tuck your chin all the way, lift your head off the ground about an inch and hold it there. Use a timer to test how long you can hold your head there without un-tucking your chin or shaking. Once you have a baseline time, do 8 repetitions of that time each day and monitor your times as they begin to improve. You should aim to hold for 35 seconds without losing form or shaking.

Other considerations for those suffering from neck pain shoud include sleeping positions, pillows used, working postures and the condition of the upper back.

Pectorals

Many of us have tight pectorals. It is particularly common among hairstylists because you work hard holding your arms up and in front of you. Tight pectorals can lead to discomfort themselves, but it's also very important to consider the effect tight pectorals have on your overall posture. If the muscles are tight, they drag your shoulders forward, your upper back down and strain your neck. This can contribute to shoulder conditions, more strains and even headaches. So stretch those pecs!!! Use B-5 and B-6.

Using the acuball to work out tension in the muscles is very effective (though unpleasant) with B-33.

Try to incorporate a good 3 minute pectoral stretch into your daily routine. This paired with exercises for your upper back muscles will ensure good posture and better working biomechanics.

Anterior Shoulder

Crossing this area is a combination of several commonly strained muscles: the anterior deltoids, the biceps, and the two pectoral muscles. Sometimes problems with rotator cuff muscles can also manifest here. It is important to seek a proper diagnosis and treatment if you experience severe sharp pains in the shoulder, weakness, pain when sleeping on the arm, or other unusual symptoms.

It will help to keep the major muscles of the area well stretched. The following stretches are designed to offset the strains you experience as a stylist. They are best done as frequently as possible, before work, after work and even during breaks at work.

Try B-5, B-6, A-9, B-4 and A-13.

With a group of muscles used as extensively as these, stretching is useful but it is also important to strengthen the antagonist muscles - the opposing muscles that move the arm and shoulder backwards. Doing so will ensure there is a balance of strength from front to back, which is quite important for joints like the shoulder that have such a large open range of motion. Use exercises B-2, B-7 and B-8.

Anterior Forearm

With the extensive use of your wrist flexor muscles, you are bound to experience tightness and pain at some point. Taking a moment to stretch these muscles in this prayer pose as often as you can when at work can do wonders (C-8). It would be ideal to do this stretch for 30 seconds every hour. When this stretch is not enough, self-massage with an acuball is helpful (C-18). For a more intense stretch, put your hand against a wall at eye level with the fingers down and the palm all the way against the wall (C-9). While keeping your elbow straight, use your other thumb to push firmly into the various tender points along the forearm and slowly massage with as much pressure as you can tolerate (C-11). Start at the inside of the elbow and work down to the wrist. Do not do this if it produces sharp pains in your wrist. If the pain is frequent and significant, or if you have any numbness or tingling in fingers, consult the next chapter on carpal tunnel syndrome, pronator teres syndrome and golfers elbow.

Knees

In a nutshell, knee pain can be the result either of injuries, imbalances or arthritis (degeneration). When managing an injury or suspecting arthritis, you are always best under the care of a doctor. Conditions that contribute to knee pain among hairstylists include poor footwear, hard floors, long working hours without breaks, extra body weight, previous knee injuries and dietary insufficiencies.

Increasing the strength of your thigh muscles will decrease knee pain, as will increasing the diversity of your activities. The best option is to learn a leg workout in the gym under the guidance of a qualified trainer or physiotherapist. Having strong gluteal muscle and strong quadriceps can decrease the occurrence and severity of knee pain.[2, 3] The stronger the muscles of your legs are, the more they bear the weight and the less force goes through the cartilage of the knees. You can increase the strength of this set of muscles significantly in as little as two months if you set your mind to it. Perform the five exercises: F-2, F-3, F-4, F-5 and

F-32 every three days. Do them each (except for F-32) at a cadence of 5 seconds down and 5 seconds up (that's very slow and takes a lot of discipline), and aim to achieve complete muscle failure at 6-8 reps. Even though it may seem counter-intuitive to take on more knee-straining activity, taking on a new challenge, like yoga, Tai Chi, a gym routine, or a new sport will almost always improve the condition of your knees.

Pain in your knees can also sometimes be the result of a problem elsewhere in your body (feet, ankles, hip or pelvis), much more commonly than most realize in fact. If your pelvis is un-level for instance (also more common than you may think), one knee will experience more rotation, weight and strain than the other. Make sure to bring up anything about your ankles, hips, or low back when you see a specialist. For knee problems I recommend a chiropractor, physiotherapist, osteopath or sports medicine practitioner.

The following forms of self-treatment are best done gently. If your pain doesn't improve within 6 weeks of improved footwear and self-treatments, see a specialist.

Begin with a mobilization which decompresses the knee (G-13). With the cylindrical object wedged right under your knee, pull back on your ankle as though you were stretching your quads. Hold the tension just for a couple seconds and repeat 30 times.

Find the popliteus muscle. Do this by running your thumb along the front of the tibia (the main shin bone) until you are near the top and stop right as it begins to flare out. Then roll your finger inwards about an inch. It will be tender when pressed on firmly. Now apply firm pressure with your thumb while you extend your leg *all* the way until it is completely strait (G-14). Continue to hold the pressure while you bend and straighten the leg 10 times. If it is most tender with a straight leg you are doing it correctly.

Lie on your side on top of a foam roller and move up and down to release the tension all along the side of your thigh (F-6). Try to keep the leg relatively strait while you roll.

Hips

As one of the most robust joints in our body, pain in our hips must be taken seriously. The material in this section is meant to help those with tight hip capsules and minor imbalances from one side to the other. These recommendations will benefit those with occasional sharp pains, soreness or stiffness in the hips. For more chronic or serious issues, refer to the conditions section of the book and seek help from a professional.

Try this:

Lying on your back with your knees bent, turn your affected hip inwards, trying to get your knee close to the ground. Use your other leg to add pressure (F-7).

Compare the range of motion of each hip in this position to the other. Spend more time doing this mobilization on the hip with less motion. Then graduate to the more challenging and very effective F-30 active mobilization. Do it at least once each day.

Then use positions F-8, F-9 and F-10 to release tension in your hips.

Stretch your gluteus medius (F-12) and hip flexors (F-10 or F-11).

Strengthening your gluteus medius muscles will directly benefit the condition of your hips. Use this side-lying glut medius exercise (F-13) to get them fired up quickly. F-3 and F-32 are great exercises that will help to round out your strengthening efforts.

Once you are ready for a more advance exercise, use a thick Theraband around your knees to increase the activation of your gluteus medius muscles while you squat (F-14).

Hamstrings

A minor strain of the hamstring is best treated with rest, elevation and compression. If not severe it will typically resolve on it's own. Avoid stretching for the first two days and avoid aggravating it with intense activity for six days to expedite the healing. Dealing with a chronic (persisting for months) hamstring strain is a matter of strengthening and lengthening. Stretch, stretch, stretch (F-15, F-16, F-17), avoid high heels for at least a month and then stretch some more. It is very important to stretch the hip flexor muscles (F-10, F-11) along with the hamstrings. This is because tight flexors increase the tension on the hamstrings.

As soon as possible (as soon as it's not painful), begin eccentric hamstring training with F- 18. Perform the hip airplane exercise with good form, 10 times each day. This will drastically improve the (eccentric) strength of the hamstrings. If you were to do just one stretch/exercise to improve your hamstrings, it should be this one.

Once you've noted progress in the hamstrings, start working on your abdominal strength (H- 1, H-2, H-3, H-5, H-6), learn how to tilt your pelvis and hold it in a posteriorly tilted position.

If your progress stretching the muscles is not sufficient, consider finding a chiropractor or physiotherapist who does PNF (Proprioceptive Neuromuscular Facilitation) stretching, MRT (Muscle Release Therapy) and kinesiology taping. For more severe and chronic injuries, seek out a therapist who provides Shockwave Therapy (TM) or a sports physician who can offer PRP injections.

Low back - General

Considering the complexity of the lower back, I recommend those with pain in the area to try the suggestions laid out here first, if relief is not found then consult the next chapter on specific conditions. If you have pain in a very specific spot, refer to the diagram on page 64. If you suffer from general pain or soreness all around your low back, you are in the right place.

Keep in mind that the stronger your core and gluteal muscles are, the less force is transmitted through the joints of your back. Therefore chronic or recurrent low back pain is best managed long-term by working on your core and strengthening your gluteals. Take ownership of your pain, stop looking for external solutions or 'cures' and start working to improve your body from the inside out. It is also worth noting that there are many misconceptions about the ideal ways to improve your core muscles.

Traditional sit-ups for instance are very hard on your spine and contribute very little to building practical core strength. Take a look at the abdominal crunch depicted in H-2. A sit-up can be more effective if done with slow contractions with the shoulders just an inch or so off the floor.

It is more valuable to train core muscles to be quick and have endurance than to work towards power. Doing front and side planks, the dead bug exercise (H-1), endurance crunches (H-2) and the 'stir the pot' exercise (H-5) will significantly improve your core and will certainly reduce your back pain (proportional to the gains you make with the exercises).

To further reduce the effects of spinal compression

(from standing all day), do a knee to chin stretch (E-1) and try a gentle rotational low back stretch (E-2).

To strengthen the gluteals, begin with F-2 and F-3 and work up to F-18/19 and F-32.

Do the following stretches each hour when you are standing all day. It's better if you can manage to do them even more frequently.

After four weeks, begin E-3, E-4, F-12 & F-10

Since your tissues thrive with a diversity of movement, the significant therapeutic value to having massages and other forms of body work done is easy to understand. If your discomfort comes about progressively throughout the day and is worse after extended bouts of standing or sitting, then it's a good bet that your tissues need more movement. Your first stop should be to visit a therapist (try a registered massage therapist, chiropractor or osteopath). Having such a treatment can offer you an important head start in your journey towards eliminating pain. It doesn't hurt to be under regular care of a competent professional either, they can help identify problems before they manifest in pain.

There are a number of useful tools to help with back soreness and pain. Take a look at the Helpful Tools section for more.

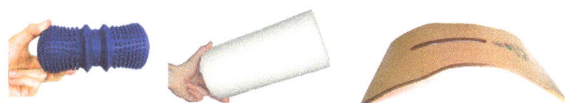

These aren't the only good tools. You can get creative using tennis balls, golf balls, old sheets, pipe, rolls of paper towel, etc.

Pelvic tilting is a valuable 'skill' to develop for those with low back pain. Tilting your pelvis forward increases the curve of your low back and tilting your pelvis backwards decreases it. This is relevant for two reasons; constantly tilting your pelvis back and forward decreases the strain of the tissues in your low back without interrupting your work. Learning to hold the pelvis in a posteriorly tilted position can help reduce symptoms caused by too much spinal compression and nerve impingement (like in sciatica). Holding the pelvis in an anteriorly tilted position can also help reduce symptoms of disc herniations or disc bulges. Therefore practicing tilting your pelvis as frequently as possible is beneficial regardless of the source of your discomfort.

Rules for chronic low back pain sufferers:

• **Stretch 5 minutes each hour**

• **Do core exercises**

• **Learn to tilt your pelvis forwards and backwards, then practice**

• **Seek out a good therapist and get treated regularly (even when not in pain)**

Notice that 3 of the 4 rules are about what you do, and only one is about having something done to you. This is important because nobody can cure your back pain for you; no chiropractor, no surgeon, no pharmacist, no physical therapist, not even that aunt you have with a penchant for magical self-cures. Your back pain is the product of your movements, your habits, the condition of your muscles, your eating habits, sleeping habits, etc. Although therapies, drugs and surgeries may help, they contribute only in part to your recovery, your efforts must constitute the bulk of the changes made. Your physical well-being is in your hands and how well you feel is proportional to how much effort you invest in optimizing it.

SI joint - Reduce pain here by stretching your gluteus medius and piriformis muscles on both sides (F-12). You can often relieve a great deal of SI pain by lying on your back with your knees bent and an acuball under your sacrum (E-14). Do the relaxing cat- camel maneuver (H-6) several times a day, and stretch the hip flexor of the opposite side of the pain (F-10) (eg. if your left SI hurts, stretch your right hip flexor)

The following exercises are also helpful:
E-5, E-6 or E-7, E-8 and E-9

QL muscle - This large deep muscle in your back works to bend you side-to-side. When it gets tense, stretch either standing up or lying down (E-3 or E-2). Use an Acuball or tennis ball directly under the tender point of the muscle (E-10), shift your weight to be as much on top of the ball as possible, keep your knees bent. Relax, take 4 very slow deep breaths and wait

at least 45 seconds. Your discomfort should dissipate along with the tension. Do this twice a day for a week.

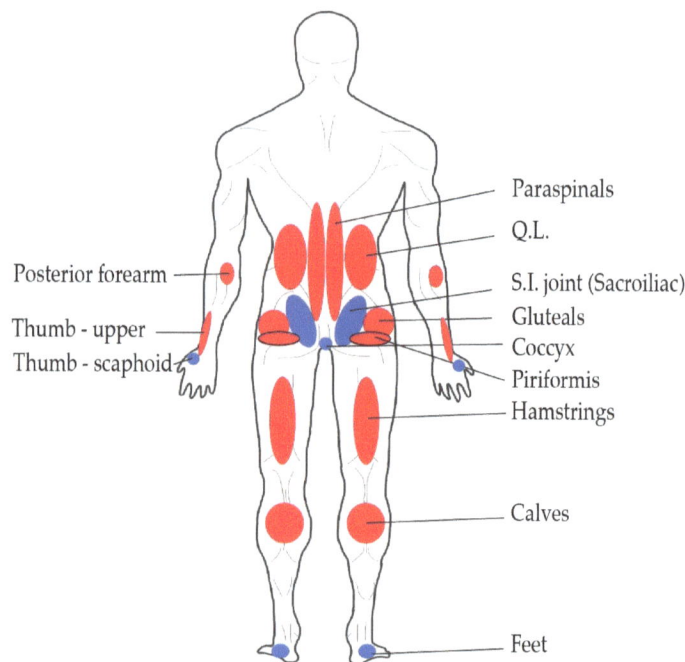

Paraspinals
Q.L.
Posterior forearm
S.I. joint (Sacroiliac)
Thumb - upper
Gluteals
Thumb - scaphoid
Coccyx
Piriformis
Hamstrings
Calves
Feet

Paraspinals - Learning to tilt your pelvis posteriorly will help reduce the strain that builds up in these muscles. Relaxing these muscles can be accomplished with many different stretches and exercises. I recommend the following: H-6, E-1, E-11, F-12, F-10, E-2

Piriformis - Pain in this area can correspond with sciatic symptoms (pain shooting down the back of your leg). To help relieve the symptoms, try these two positions: E-12, F-20

Stretch the piriformis muscles regularly with these moves: F-12, F-21, F-22, F-23

Gluteals - These commonly overworked muscles are generally robust but can cause problems when one side is holding more tension than the other. Stretch the muscles (F-12) and use techniques F-6, F-29 and F-23 to reduce tension on the problematic side.

Coccyx - If you have pain here in the coccyx, it is likely from a bump or fall. Otherwise you may be experiencing ligament strain from tight gluteal muscles (see above). If it is tender to the touch and hurts to sit, you may have damaged the cartilage or bone and it's best to see your doctor. Beyond getting yourself a donut cushion to sit on, there aren't too many helpful self-administered therapies.

Calves

Your calves are very robust muscles, though it is still quite possible to strain them. The most common cause of painful or strained calves is a bout of extreme activity (tennis, calf workout, sprinting, jumping). If that's the

case, resting and icing your leg should be sufficient and a minor strain should resolve within a few days. Calf pain that comes on slowly and gets worse while you work most likely has to do with poor footwear or a leg asymmetry. As a caution, if you are over 50 or have a history of vascular issues, see your doctor to rule out deep vein thrombosis (a medical condition where a blood clot in the leg causes calf pain).

Wearing heels shortens the calf muscles and leads to increased tension. Unsupportive shoes can also lead to straining certain parts of the calves more than the other and should be dealt with before the changes become chronic. For further guidance, consult the chapter on choosing good footwear. Since they are always active, calves are particularly susceptible to cramping. For help managing muscle cramping, see the section on it in the next chapter. If you suffer persistent cramping in just one leg and suspect a leg length difference, seek treatment from your chiropractor or osteopath.

Choose your preferred method of calf stretching among G-1, G-9 and G-10. To further lengthen a stubbornly tight calf, use the acuball mini (G-11) or foam roller (G-12) to reduce the tension in the muscle.

Feet

Sore feet are mistreated feet. Make a few changes to your footwear, spend a few minutes a day working on your feet and you should have happy feet in no time.

Cushioned insoles are a good thing, I recommend using them. No amount of cushion however can make up for a shoe without adequate support. Assess the quality of your shoe (refer to 'Choosing Good Footwear' chapter), wear cushioned insoles, consider custom orthotics and if you haven't found the perfect shoe then alternate your footwear daily (only necessary if you get sore feet). Then use the following techniques to treat yourself: G-2, G-3, G-4, G-5

Strengthening the small muscles of the foot will help reduce muscle soreness (G-6). Lay a towel flat on the ground and pick it up off the ground with your foot 15 times every other day. Single leg calf raises done at a very slow pace (G-7) and drawing the (invisible) alphabet with your foot (G-8) are exercises that will also improve the overall condition of your feet.

Note: If you are dealing with issues like bunions, plantar fasciitis, sprains or another condition, consult the advice in the next chapter and seek the help of a professional. Podiatrists are typically the best option for foot problems.

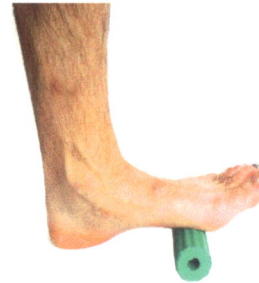
G - 2

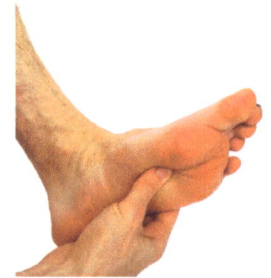
G - 4

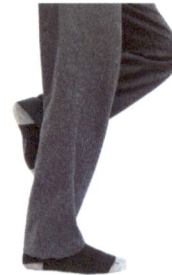
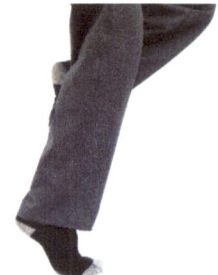
G - 7

2. J. E. Earl, and A. Z. Hoch, "A Proximal Strengthening Program Improves Pain, Function, and Biomechanics in Women with Patellofemoral Pain Syndrome," American Journal of Sports Medicine 39 (2011): 154–63.
3. K. Khayambashi et al., "The Effects of Isolated Hip Abductor and External Rotator Muscle Strengthening on Pain, Health Status, and Hip Strength in Females with Patellofemoral Pain: a Randomized Controlled Trial," Journal of Orthopaedic and Sports Physical Therapy 42 (2012): 22–29.

Other Helpful Tips

When managing pain in general, it is valuable to consider variables beyond the specific area that contribute to your condition.

Sleep quality and duration will have an impact on your ability to heal and on the way you experience pain. Take a look at the chapter on sleep later in the book. Taking measures to enhance sleep will bring about a wide range of health improvements.

Nutrition plays a big role in your ability to resolve inflammation (most painful conditions involve inflammation). Reduce your intake of pro-inflammatory foods that are fried, fatty or high in sugar. Increase you intake of natural anti-inflammatory foods like ginger, turmeric and fish oils. A dietician, nutritionist or naturopath can be very helpful.

Exercise can be very therapeutic, especially when struggling with pain or an injury. Exercising releases your built in pain-killing endorphins. So get moving, but make sure to start with forms of exercise you are comfortable with. Generally, the more intense the exercise, the more endorphins are released.

Re-wire your brain. That's right! Leading neuroscientists have helped us understand that we have much more control over how our body operates and how we experience pain than we ever thought before. For those in chronic pain frustrated with all that they've tried, I highly recommend picking up two brilliant books written by Norman Doidge on neuroplasticity; 'The Brain that Changes Itself' and 'The Brain's Way of Healing'.

Seek treatment from a therapist you trust. The suggested forms of therapy included in this chapter are but a sampling of the options out there for you. People typically get the most relief from therapies that they are comfortable with and that they believe in. Whether it is laser therapy, meditation training, cognitive behavioral therapy, energy therapy, ultrasound, Thai massage, Chinese cupping or hydrotherapy, you can benefit a great deal from a wide variety of therapeutic approaches.

7

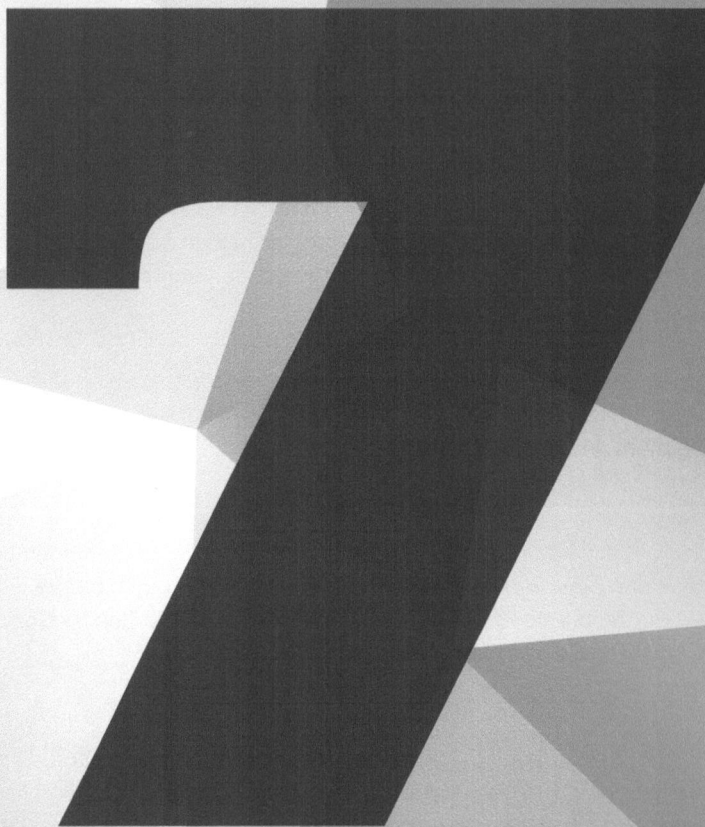

Remember, the information in this chapter is meant to better inform you and offer you guidance for a diagnosed condition. I share the best techniques for self-care and some conservative (non-surgical) treatment options. Though useful, this advice is meant to supplement the diagnosis and care of a health care professional, rather than replace it. If you are experiencing serious symptoms of any kind, or your symptoms are not getting better, you should certainly seek care.

Specific Injuries & Conditions

"It is a capital mistake to theorize before one has data. Insensibly one begins
to twist facts to suit theories, instead of theories to suit facts."

- Sir Arthur Conan Doyle

Hands

Carpal Tunnel Syndrome (CTS) is one of the most commonly misdiagnosed (and self- diagnosed) conditions around. If you suspect you have CTS, it is important to seek a proper diagnosis and treatment. The symptoms are typically numbness, tingling and pain in the thumb and first three fingers. Symptoms can also include a weakened grip or progressing 'clumsiness', night pain and stiffness.

The carpal bones - the bones in the wrist - create a 'U shape' protective barrier for the nerves, blood vessels and tendons of your arm to pass through. The 'U' is topped off by a thick piece of ligament. When there is swelling in the wrist, or if the space inside becomes narrowed for any other reason, the susceptible median nerve gets compressed, causing the symptoms. During pregnancy or even during menses, the body's tissues tend to retain more fluid which can contribute to this space being narrowed. Constant pressure on the wrists (like using a keyboard) and certain repetitive movements can also lead to the compression of this space and of the median nerve. Vibration also contributes to the worsening of the condition. If the wrist is held bent backwards or forwards while you use scissors, a brush or a dryer, you may be adding extra compression to the carpal tunnel. You may be particularly susceptible to developing CTS if you

have had a previous injury to the area, if you wear tight watches or bracelets, if you have diabetes, are overweight, have thyroid dysfunction or are pregnant.[4]

TIP: Sleeping with your wrists bent (and therefore compressed) is often an overlooked cause or aggravator of CTS

Self-test: Perform the stretch C-13 (pictured below) for 2 minutes. If this produces a burning sensation, numbness and tingling in the fingers or clumsiness, it is a positive test. Visit your family doctor, who will likely send you for an EMG nerve conduction test.

If you have any numbness or tingling, it is important that you seek a diagnosis even if the self-test is negative. You can also visit a sports physician, chiropractor, or have your family doctor refer you to a neurologist.

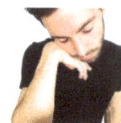

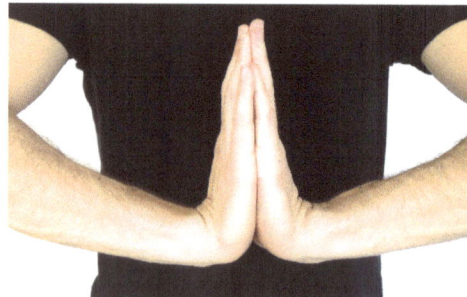

SUGGESTED TREATMENT

SHORT TERM

Reduce workload temporarily as best you can. When the wrists are aggravated, it is wise to rest and avoid the activities that exacerbate it. Pay really close attention to the movements of your affected wrist while you work and modify your shoulder and wrist ergonomics; consult the 'Optimal Biomechanics' section of this book.

Have a therapist massage the neck, shoulder, arm, forearm, wrist and hand. Have three subsequent massages within two weeks.

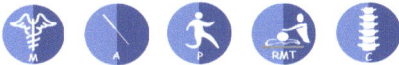

Consider wearing a wrist brace. They may be cumbersome, but are often only necessary for a short time. If you are in significant pain and need to make immediate changes, it may be a good option. It will serve to minimize any problematic or aggravating movements of the wrist. Any standard drug store or medical equipment supply store will carry wrist braces for carpal tunnel. The particular brand or features make little difference.
If you sleep with your wrist(s) bent, wear a wrist brace to bed for 1-3 weeks and take account of any changes that it may make.

Perform the following stretches as frequently as possible in between activities at work: C-12, C-13, C-28

Perform the following stretches twice a day at home: C-9, C-14, C-15

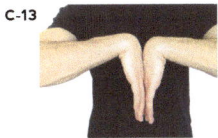

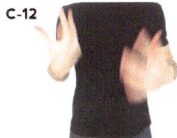

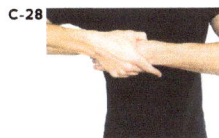

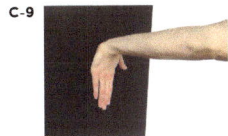

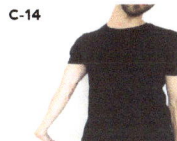

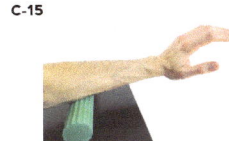

C-13   C-12   C-28

C-9   C-14   C-15

Full descriptions of stretches are in Exercise Appendix

LONG TERM

Ergonomic tips for CTS

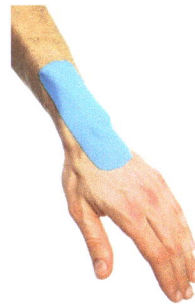

Identify any movements that take the wrist out of neutral repetitively and figure out a way to change the need to perform that movement. You can buy kinesiology tape and wear a single strip on the backside of your wrist to help with this. Use wrist or forearm support when using a computer. Massage the muscles of the forearm. Apply cold when it is first aggravated, and alternate heat and cold if it has become chronic.

Stretch the fingers, wrists, forearms, shoulder and neck before starting to work. Stretch for 1- 5 minutes every hour of work. Treatments that help include massage, chiropractic, physiotherapy, acupuncture and osteopathy. If you have symptoms that are continuing to get worse despite trying management protocols described above, seek the opinion of your family doctor who will likely refer you to a specialist for a surgical consultation.

Like in most cases, the surgery should be considered only after less-invasive options have proven ineffective.

Supplementing with vitamin B6 (100mg/TID for 2-3 months), vitamin C & bioflavinoids and bromalain has been shown to improve the outcome of CTS [5, 6]

The following have also been known to benefit the outcome of the condition: Coenzyme Q10 & coenzyme A - 30-90mg daily (improves tissue oxygenation) Lecithin - 1200mg 3 times daily, before meals (aides nerve function). Zinc - 50mg daily (enhances healing)

Rehabilitation Early stage
Perform nerve flossing of the median nerve C-14 as well as A-13 and C-18

Rehabilitation Late stage
D-1 and C-36

Hands

Pronator teres syndrome is a condition that presents similarly to carpal tunnel syndrome. It happens when the median nerve is compressed in-between the two heads of the pronator teres muscle in the forearm rather than in the carpal tunnel. The muscle turns your hand inwards (doing the 'thumbs-down' action), and if it is overused it can become tight. This tightness closes the space where the median nerve travels through and causes shooting pain, tingling and other symptoms into your hand.

Dealing with a pronator teres problem entails reducing the tension in the muscle, and then undoing the habit that lead to its development. The first part is the easy part; stretch the muscle and massage it regularly.

Everyone's movement patterns are quite unique, so you'll have to pay close attention to discover how you've been straining this muscle. If you are unable to resolve your symptoms by self-treating or making small changes to your activities, then seek the guidance of a specialist.

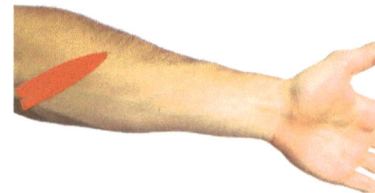

The location of the pronator teres

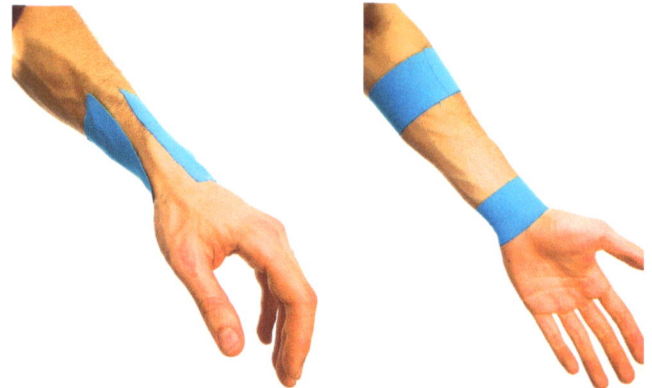

Two possible kinesiology tape applications that would be helpful to prevent overuse of the muscle

SUGGESTED TREATMENT

SHORT TERM

Turn the wrist so the thumb moves as far clockwise as you can go, and straighten your elbow, pushing your palm into the table/wall. Then use your thumb to dig into tender points (tender = tight) and swipe along the line shown with as much pressure as is tolerated (C-16).

C-16

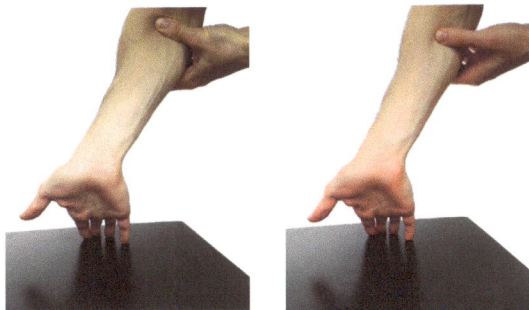

Roll out the tension in the muscles at least once a day for 8 days; C-18

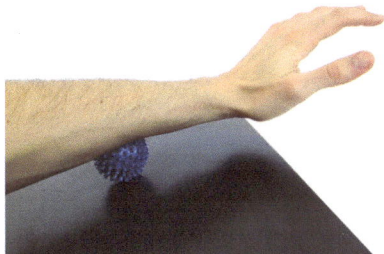

C-18

Full descriptions of stretches can be found in the in Exercise Appendix

LONG TERM

Ergonomic tips for CTS

Stretch the whole group of forearm muscles daily: C-8, C-11, C-17

Continue to use the acuball mini to massage the muscles of the forearm if the tension isn't yet resolved: C-18. Use this technique for up to 21 days.

C-8

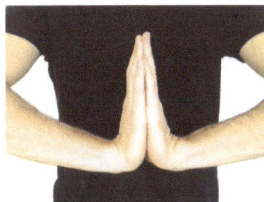

C-17

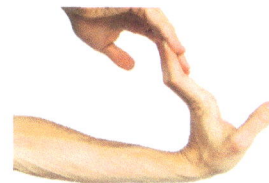

C-11

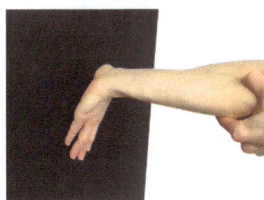

C-11

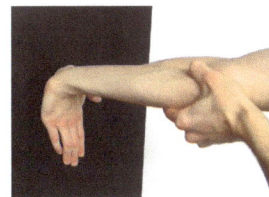

Rehabilitation Early stage
See the kinesiology tape application for pronator teres either on the previous page or in the exercise appendix: C-19

Rehabilitation Late stage
Use a Theraband flexbar to eccentrically rehabilitate the forearm wrist flexor muscles; C-26

While working, practice minimizing excessive wrist movements. Keep wrist movements to a minimum by compensating with your elbow and shoulder.

Hands

DeQuervain's Tenosynovitis is an issue that many hairstylists struggle with. It is a condition in which the tendons of two muscles in the forearm become irritated from overuse. Aggravating movements include extending your thumb outwards (as you would when opening scissors), and rotating or tilting the wrist towards your pinky. The condition is characterized by pain on the thumb side of the forearm, just above the wrist. The two muscles are named extensor pollicis brevis and abductor pollicis longus. They start at your elbow as muscle and narrow into tendon they get closer to your wrist and attach on bones in your hand. Their primary job is to bring the wrist and the thumb up and back, as in a 'thumb's up' position. When these small muscles are worked too hard, they get tight and the tendon starts to get inflamed* and painful from all the friction.

*Nerd alert! Although inflammation is a useful way to understand the problem, technically it isn't actually inflammation in the tendon, rather it's something called peritendinous fibrosis and fibrocartilaginous metaplasia of the tendon sheath tissue.[7] This bit of knowledge might help to explain why taking anti-inflammatories won't help much with the symptoms in this case.

Self test: If you have DeQuervain's Tenosynovitis, you will have pain along the thumb side of your arm, concentrated mostly in the area along the wrist. A quick way to confirm that this is your issue is by doing the following test. Tuck your thumb into your fist as much as you can and then tilt your fist down towards the pinky (C-20).

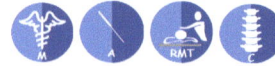

C-20

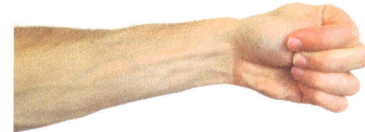

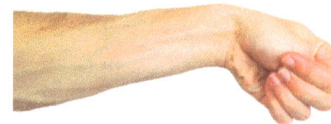

SELF TEST FOR DEQUERVAINS TENOSYNOVITIS

SUGGESTED TREATMENT

SHORT TERM

Using a wrist support or an application of kinesiology tape will prove very useful in minimizing the aggravation while you recover. While reducing the stress on the tendon, you can work to resolve the tension of the muscles that pull on it. An uncomfortable but effective self-treatment for the extensor carpi radialis should be done daily (C-21). The same should be done with the muscle called the brachioradialis, as demonstrated in C-24.

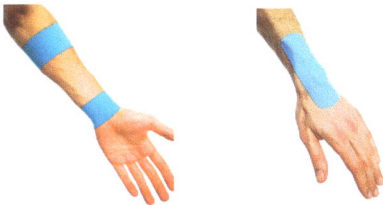

These active stretches are best done in sets of 6, once or twice a day

C-21

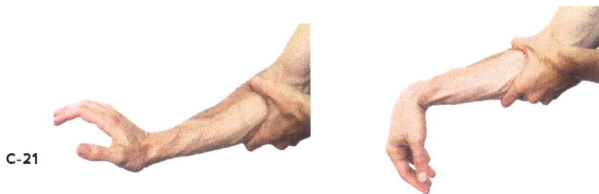

C-24

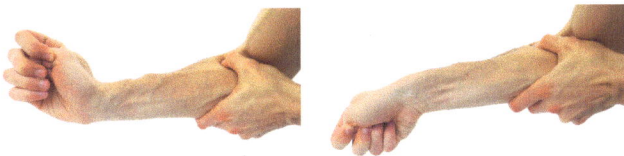

Full descriptions of stretches are in Exercise Appendix

LONG TERM

Continue to more advanced stretching of the wrist extensor muscles

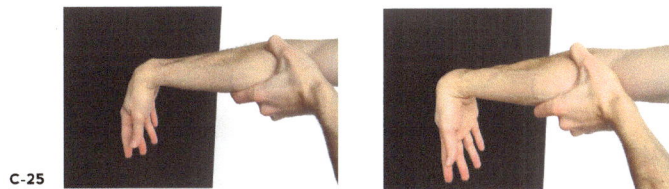

C-25

Rehabilitation Early stage
Modifying the aggravating activities is crucial. Consult the chapter on optimal biomechanics, use kinesiology tape for two weeks to enhance position sense in the arm and alternate your hand positions when cutting, drying, brushing or coloring.

Rehabilitation Late stage
Train the group of forearm muscles eccentrically with a theraband flexbar (C-23)
Begin eccentric training of pronation with theraband (C-26)

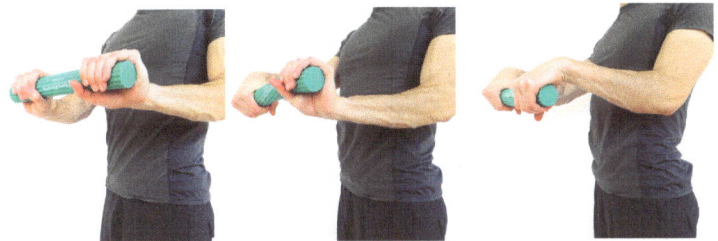

Hands

Ganglion cysts are more common among hairstylists than in the general population because of the amount of repetitive strain on your wrists. Ganglion cysts are fluid filled bulges in tendon sheaths in the wrist. They *can* develop spontaneously but are usually associated with extensive and repetitive finger movements. They most often appear here:

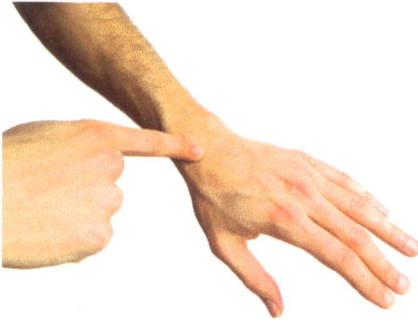

They are only painful sometimes, they often come back even after being removed and can sometimes (but rarely) cause numbness and tingling in the fingers.

If a ganglion cyst is not painful (or seldom painful) and doesn't interfere with the use of your hand, it is usually safe to leave it without doing anything. For symptomatic ganglions, you can tape a button over it to apply pressure up to 3 weeks. Although this can work, there is a high likelihood that it will come back.

In the past, people were often advised to thump the ganglion with a bible or heavy object to get rid of it. It is risky and not recommended! (you can rupture and damage tissues. Not to mention it's not very effective).

Note that ganglion cysts can become aggravated when pregnant or when menstruating. This is because the hormones released in the body during this time cause increased fluid retention, causing the ganglions to temporarily expand.

SUGGESTED TREATMENT

SHORT TERM

Place a button on the cyst and tape it down with moderate pressure - enough to apply continuous pressure but not so much as to impact circulation of blood to the hands.

Have a therapist treat the muscles of your forearm. Or you can work out the tension yourself with C-11, C-15, C-29, C-21 and C-25

Have kinesiology tape applied to your wrist and forearm professionally. The movement of the muscles and bones in your wrist have a significant impact on ganglion cysts. Regardless of whether or not problematic movements caused it, an improvement in the coordination of your wrist movements will help.

C-23

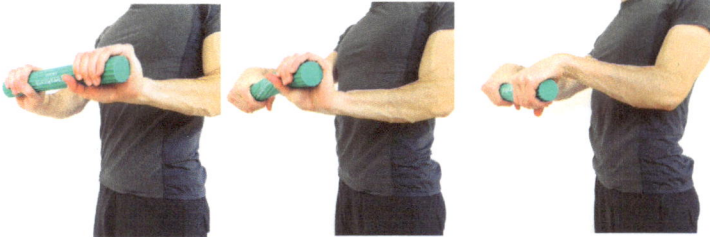

C-30

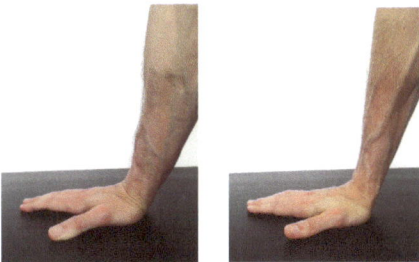

LONG TERM

Unless you are content tolerating it, continue to explore various treatment options. Ultrasound therapy, cold laser therapy and acupuncture have varying levels of efficacy and are worth a try if your cyst persists.

It is possible to have a ganglion removed surgically, which has a 5-15% chance of returning. Visit your family doctor for a referral if appropriate.[8]

C-28

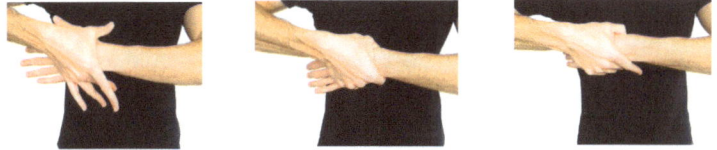

C-25

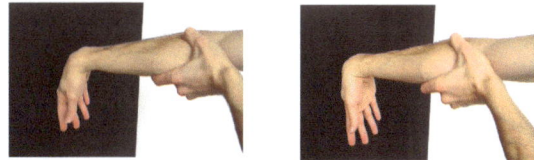

Rehabilitation Early stage
In the earlier stages of healing, use exercises C-28 & C-25

Rehabilitation Late stage
After 3-4 weeks, begin with C-23 & C-30

Full descriptions of stretches are in Exercise Appendix

Hands

Trigger finger & trigger thumb can develop over time with extensive use of scissors. It is defined by the tendency for a finger/thumb to get stuck in a bent position, and the subsequent inability to fully straighten the digit without pain, a 'snap' or both. To understand what's happening, imagine a train going back and forth through a tunnel. Imagine what would happen if you put a big pile of rubbish on the train tracks right at the entrance to the tunnel. The train would have to squeeze through the tunnel over the pile of rubbish, and once it did it would have a hard time coming back the other way too. Trigger finger is the result of tissue buildup or swelling (called a nodule) around the tendon that moves your finger, causing trouble for the tendon moving through the sheath. It can develop as a result of overuse, but can also be associated with osteoarthritis, rheumatoid arthritis or an injury to the tendon. [9]

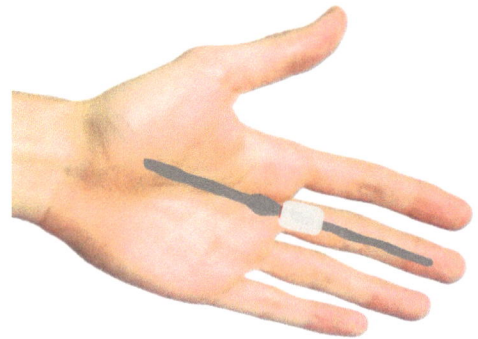

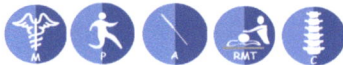

SUGGESTED TREATMENT

SHORT TERM

Begin by resting the hand for three days. Then, if possible tape the affected finger to the adjacent finger (keeping it straight) for 5 days.

Do the C-9, C-31 and C-32 stretches three times each day for two minutes each time.

Rehabilitation Early stage

Use the Handmaster exercise ball or a Power Web to strengthen the muscles that keep the fingers elongated. Train all five fingers at once and train the affected finger alone as well. Using a mild to moderate level of resistance, perform a total of 50 repetitions each day for the first 2 weeks,

then 30 repetitions each day for the following 4 weeks.

LONG TERM

Avoid excessive pinching and gripping for three weeks. Avoid vibrating tools (electric clippers for instance) as much as possible. If no progress is made after 12 weeks of self-treatment & therapy, request a consultation with a surgeon. Consider learning to use a different type of shear.

Rehabilitation Late stage

Continue strengthening the muscles that extend the fingers with ball or web.

Use an elastic band to train the muscles that separate the fingers from each other (C-33).

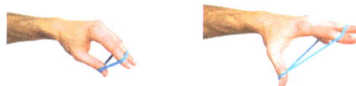

If symptoms progress or don't get any better after 4-6 weeks after using the above techniques, there are a few more aggressive treatment options to consider. Here is a review of the most effective therapies to inform your decision.

Treatment should start with first having a healthcare professional produce a diagnosis and rule out any associated or underlying issues.

Splinting is often the first option because it's easy and noninvasive (not surgical). It consists of simply wearing a splint that holds your affected finger in an elongated position to keep the tendon stretched.

Manual Therapy can be provided by a chiropractor, osteopath, physiotherapist, massage therapist or others. Treating the forearm muscles and the affected tendon, the therapist can help to mitigate the strain your tissues tolerate and you can expect progressive improvements. Tendon 'scraping' techniques like Gua Sha and Graston™ can also be effective treatments as they work to break down the extra tissue build up along the tendons. Collectively these techniques are referred to as 'tool-assisted soft tissue therapies'.

Shockwave therapy is effective but painful. It is noninvasive and often produces results relatively quickly. It is a device used by a variety of therapists that delivers an intense sonic impulse and breaks up tissue adhesions. Its positive outcomes have been demonstrated in a decent amount of research, albeit mostly in cases of calcific tendonitis (most often in the shoulder). If you seek out this therapy - which I do recommend - you should expect a minimum of 3 and maximum of 10 treatments. *N.B. It is also called 'extracorporeal shockwave therapy'.

Low Level Laser Therapy (or 'cold laser') is another very good noninvasive treatment option. Emitting a concentrated wavelength of light can help to accelerate tissue healing. Expect between 4 and 10 sessions.

A Steroid injection may be a good option[10] especially if you are experiencing a lot of pain. Corticosteroids won't directly affect the tissue build up, but can reduce inflammation and reduce pain which allows your body a better chance of healing itself.

Surgery is generally encouraged by experts if you've already tried self-care, shockwave and steroid injections all unsuccessfully. The surgery is typically successful with about a 3% recurrence rate. [11, 12, 13, 14, 15]

Arm

Muscle strains in the hand and arm are common, not surprisingly considering the excessive demand you put on them. If you experience nagging aches in tender areas of your hand or arm and you've ruled out the various conditions listed in this section, then it's likely that you have a strained muscle or two. Strained muscles will feel worse the more you work, will generally hurt in the same area (the area of pain doesn't change or move). Muscle pain is sore and achy. To help you differentiate: Nerve pain is sharp and shooting, capsule pain is pinching, sharp and specific to certain movements, and bone pain is deep and dull.

To deal with a muscle strain you must address the cause and then treat the muscle. Pay attention to the specific movements, tasks and positions that aggravate the area. Get creative and modify the way you do that activity, at least temporarily. Following the specific postural guidance in this book, you might find it useful to change the way you hold your shoulder, the height of the chair, the equipment you use or your wrist position when using it. For self-treatment techniques for specific muscles, refer to the self-treatment protocols in the Pain & How to Fix it chapter.

Note: if you follow the advice above and the problem persists or is complicated with other symptoms, seek a diagnosis and treatment from a qualified professional.

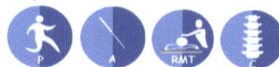

Arm

Muscle cramping can be the result of overuse, a sign of poor working postures (leading to overloading of specific muscles) or a deficiency of certain metabolites. If you are experiencing muscle cramping for the first time, it's likely that you have just overused the muscle. Rest and stretching it well will be sufficient to resolve the cramp. If the cramping is recurrent, we must consider the cause to be either consistenly poor working postures or a metabolic imbalance. While you consult the chapter in this book on Optimal Biomechanics and review your habits, try the following remedies in order until the problem is resolved*.

Magnesium (750mg daily)

Calcium (1500mg daily)

Vitamin E (200 IU daily)

Potassium (90mg daily)

Malic acid (as directed on label)

Silica (as directed on label)

Vitamin B complex (50 mg of each major B vitamin 3 times daily with meals)

Vitamin C with bioflavonoids (4000 mg daily)

Vitamin D3 (400 IU daily)

If your cramping doesn't improve within a few weeks or if it becomes worse, seek medical guidance. This is important because muscle cramping can be caused (or aggravated) by a variety of medical conditions. The list includes: vitamin E deficiency, anemia, fibromyalgia, hormone imbalances, allergies, arthritis, arteriosclerosis, dehydration, heat stroke, hypothyroidism, varicose veins and amyotrophic lateral sclerosis (Lou Gehrig's disease). Some medications can have the side effect of causing muscle cramping.[16] If you take prescription medications, ask your pharmacist about the side effects and tell your prescribing doctor about your symptoms.

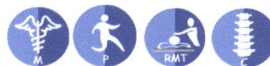

*Note: Consult your doctor before taking any supplements.

Arm

Tennis elbow (lateral epicondylitis) is a common condition that causes pain on the outside of the forearm close to the elbow. The tendon where all the posterior forearm muscles meet gets inflamed from overuse. Collectively these muscles bring the wrist up. The pain typically comes and goes, gets worse after working and can be bad in the mornings (as the inflammation accumulates and settles while you sleep).

If pressing firmly right here is intensely painful and tender..

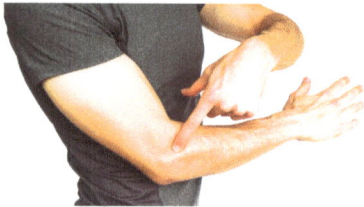

that is a strong indication that you have this issue.

It's called tennis elbow because the backhand swing in tennis is particularly strenuous for these forearm muscles. Tennis players are therefore susceptible to developing the issue (as are hairstylists).

Note: Tennis elbow is sometimes related to a shoulder problem. It is important to consider any pain or issues in the shoulders when dealing with tennis elbow.

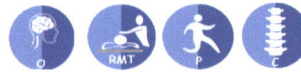

Self-Test: Stretching the arm in this position will cause discomfort when you have tennis elbow.

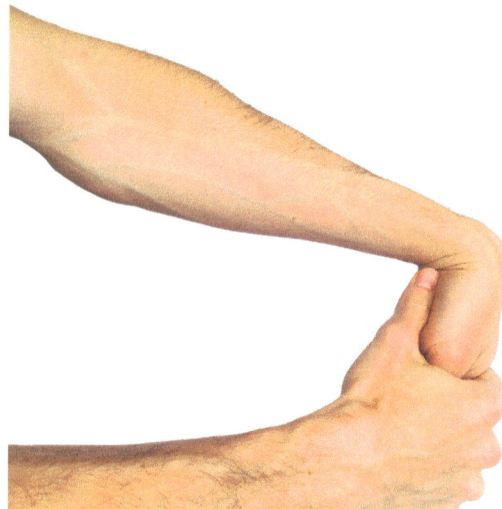

SUGGESTED TREATMENT

SHORT TERM

Treating tennis elbow can sometimes take up to several weeks, so don't be discouraged. The most important step overall will be modifying the way you use the affected wrist. Refer to the section on the wrist in the chapter on Optimal Biomechanics.

Icing the painful area (10 minutes on, 10 minutes off, 10 minutes on) in the evening will be of some help.

Self massage the posterior forearm muscles two or three times daily - C-10, C-23, C-25, C-29.

Wear a tennis elbow brace. Wear the brace for several hours a day for a minimum of two weeks. It can be a very useful tool, one I highly recommend using- but only temporarily - for a maximum of three months. Wearing it while you work reduces the strain put on the tendon. If the brace has a pressure pad (a little nubbin bumpy thing), position the bump overtop of the most tender muscle along the posterior forearm. Do not wear the brace to sleep.

Kinesiology tape in two helpful applications: on the palm side of your wrist and on the back side of the wrist. On the palm side of the wrist, the tape will help to minimize the wrist movement that causes the irritation and pain. On the back side of your wrist, the tape may serve to keep your wrist out of an excessively bent position while you sleep (addressing a factor many don't realize is at play).

Topical creams can be useful to reduce symptoms. Creams that contain capsaicin, menthol, analgesics or muscle relaxants are effective.

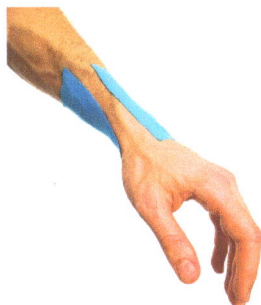

LONG TERM

It is particularly important for you to reconsider your technique using blow dryers, spin brushes and scissors.

Continue to practice the improved postures set out in the chapter on Optimal Mechanics of the wrist.

Ensure you are not bending your wrists down while you sleep. If you believe that you are, pick up a general purpose wrist guard to wear at night for a few months while you recover.

Rehabilitation Early stage
C-34 or C-35. 20 slow repetitions once a day for two weeks.

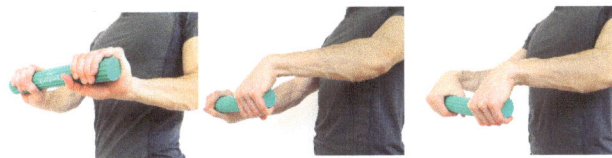

Rehabilitation Late stage
Continue C-34 or C-35 three times per week for an additional month.
Ensuring healthy arm mechanics will help reduce the strain on your forearm. Train your rotator cuff muscles with C-40 and C-41

Arm

Golfers elbow (medial epicondylitis) is essentially the same injury as tennis elbow except that it's on the other side of the forearm. It is caused by excessive use of the muscles that grasp and bend the wrist down.

Pain & tenderness will be focused at this point

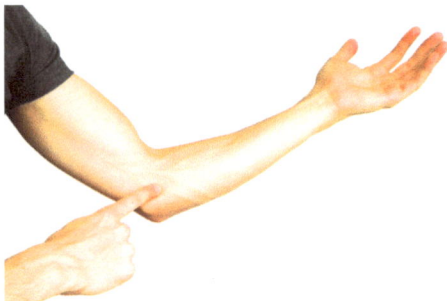

Pulling the hand and wrist back to stretch the forearm muscles will be uncomfortable when you have golfers elbow.

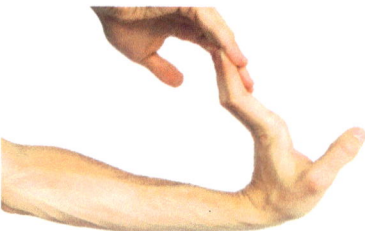

If you are afflicted with golfers elbow it is important to reassess your patterns of wrist movement with your work. Keeping the wrist too far up or too far down while you cut or comb will create extra strain on the forearm muscles.

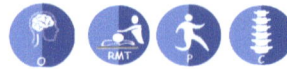

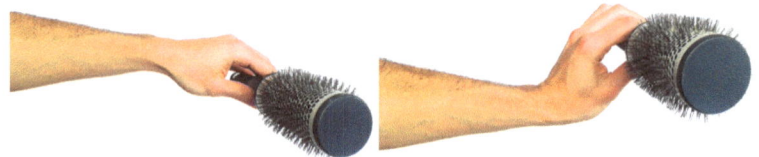

Good   **Bad**

SUGGESTED TREATMENT

SHORT TERM

Perform C-8, C-9 and C-11 3 times a day for two weeks

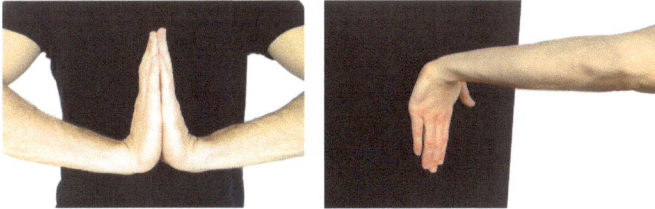

Use a golfers/tennis elbow brace (they are often the same thing) at least 80% of the time while you work. Wearing the golfers elbow brace will take the pressure off the main tendon near your elbow and allow the area to recover. However, without properly correcting your wrist movements, the problem will likely recur when you cease using the brace.

Ice just below the elbow on the inside of the forearm (10 minutes on, 10 minutes off, 10 minutes on) in the evenings for the first 10 days.

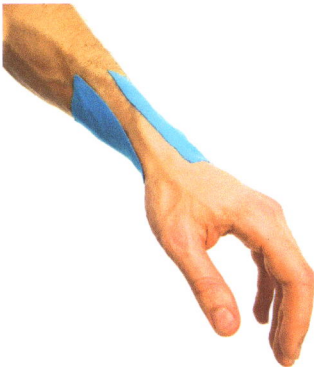

Kinesiology tape in a simple application on the underside of the forearm can be helpful to offset the strain while you work.

LONG TERM

It is particularly important for you to reconsider your technique using blow dryers, spin brushes and scissors.

Ensure you are not bending your wrists down while you sleep. If you believe that you are, pick up a general purpose wrist guard or kinesiology tape to wear at night for a few months while you recover.

Review the chapter on Optimal Biomechanics of the wrist.

Continue working on stretching and massaging the forearm muscles regularly.

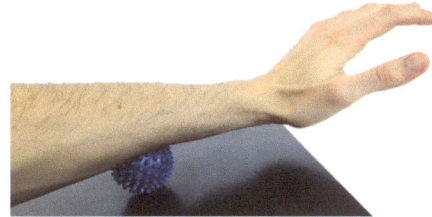

Rehabilitation Early stage
C-36 or C-37
Train the muscles that straighten the fingers with C-4.

Rehabilitation Late stage
Continue C-36 or C-37 3 times per week for a month, and begin doing C-40 and C-41 regularly.

Arm

Shoulder impingement is a common cause of sharp pain in the shoulder. It happens when you spend a lot of time working with arms up. When your arm is elevated, the space between the acromion (the bone covering the top of your shoulder) and humerus

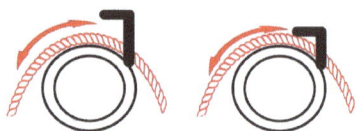

(arm bone) narrows and compresses the rotator cuff tendons. Normally the shoulder blade tilts backwards when the arm is lifted to open up the space in the shoulder for the tendons to glide through. In some cases, when a lot of time is spent working with the arms up, the muscles in the front become strong but the muscles in the back that tilt the shoulder blade don't keep up very well.

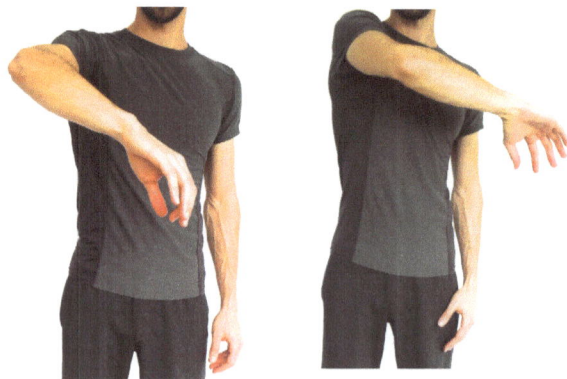

The tendons in the shoulder begin to get compressed and wear out faster. The compression is made worse with poor posture (upper back slouching and shoulders rolled forward). Putting your arm in these positions will exacerbate the pain.

The more time you spend working with your arms elevated the more pain you'll experience. The pain will often get worse at night and rolling over onto your bad shoulder will wake you up. There will be points of tenderness around the bony prominence of your shoulder and you may have pain radiating further down the front or side of your arm. If you suspect that you have an impingement issue it is important that you seek out a qualified clinician and manage your expectations - impingement is not always quick to resolve. That said, when addressed in the early stages of development, impingement issues respond very well to conservative treatment like the plan laid out on to your right.

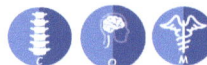

SUGGESTED TREATMENT

SHORT TERM

Ice (10 minutes on, 10 minutes off, alternating 3 times) when the shoulder is aggravated.

Begin doing pendulum exercises immediately (C-42) and shoulder blade mobilizations (B-22).

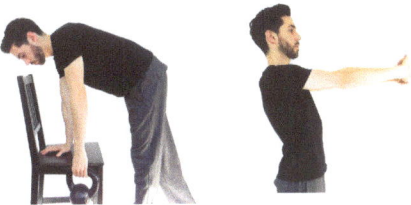

Gentle stretches for the muscles that encourage impingement are also important - B-4, B-5, B-30

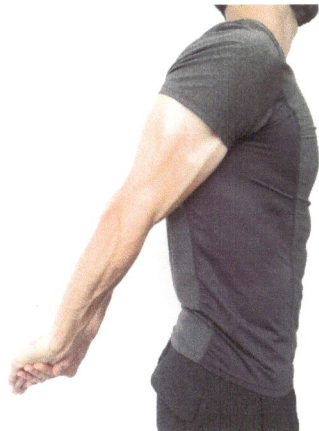

LONG TERM

Use C-43, C-47, B-13, B-17 and D-5 to balance the strength and length of the shoulder muscles.

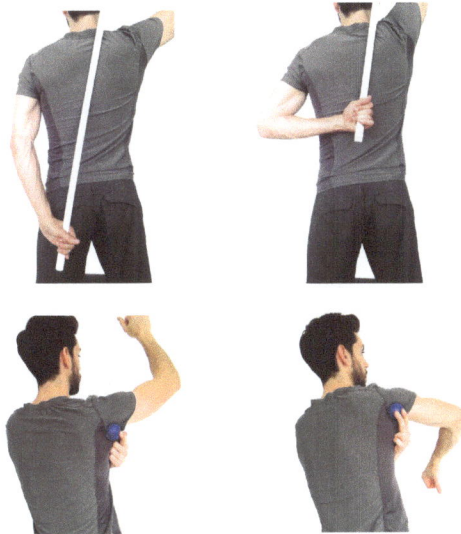

Rehabilitation Early stage
Start with C-40 and C-41. Good form is absolutely essential.

Rehabilitation Late stage
Continue onto B-1, B-2, B-8 and B-28 after 3 weeks of the previous exercises.

Arm

Rotator cuff strain

As one of the more common chronic issues experienced by hairstylists, rotator cuff strains are tough to deal with. If not dealt with properly, it is more likely that it will develop into further injury, a chronic tendon problem and eventually increase your risk of developing arthritis. The rotator cuff is comprised of the tendons of four muscles that work together to facilitate the intricate movements of the shoulder. If even just one of the muscles gets tight, short or misbehaves, the normal balanced movement of the shoulder joint is compromised.

As with most chronic injuries, the first and most difficult step of management requires changing the habits that contribute to the issue. Refer to the Optimal Biomechanics chapter of this book and work on modifying your shoulder and arm posture while you work.

Following a basic exercise program for several weeks will strengthen the muscles of the rotator cuff, reducing the extent of negative strain. The exercises and stretches together will contribute to restoring normal movement to the joint. Perform the exercises below and those under 'short term' on the next page 5 days per week, doing three sets of ten repetitions of each.

B - 1

B - 13

B-4

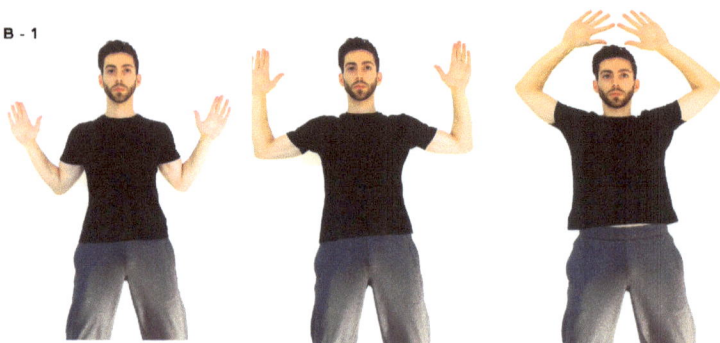
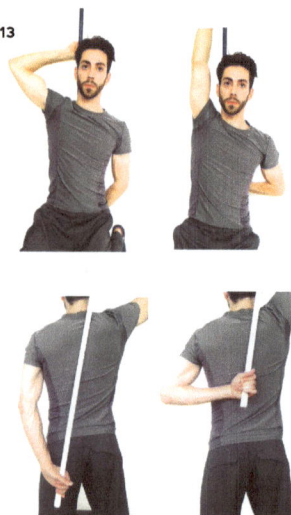
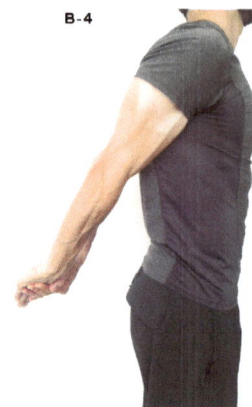

SUGGESTED TREATMENT

SHORT TERM

Ensuring NOT to take your shoulder through painful ranges of motion, perform the following exercises in a slow and controlled fashion. Together they contribute to strengthening the muscles and tendons of the rotator cuff as well as improving the coordination of shoulder movements. C-40, C-41, B-13, B-16, B-22, B-4

C-41

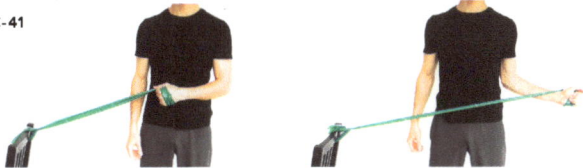

C-40

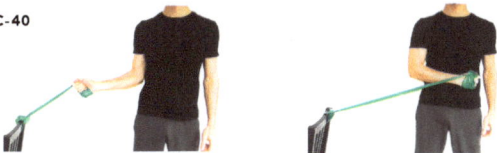

B-16

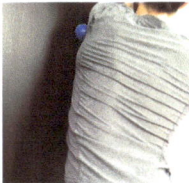

B-22

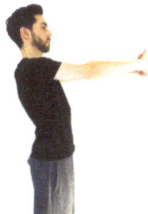

Full descriptions of exercises are in Exercise Appendix

LONG TERM

If your rotator cuff problem is recurring or getting worse despite your efforts, visit a sports physician or chiropractor to start the process of engaging in a more intensive care plan. Since 'rotator cuff strain' is somewhat of an umbrella term, encompassing dozens of possible and more specific issues, specific advice on the best therapies is limited here.

Continue with the exercises you enjoy and begin with B-25 and B-30.

Kinesiology tape applications can help to temporarily improve the movements in the shoulders. These are three good options.

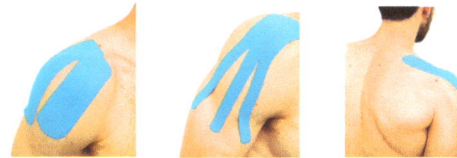

Rehabilitation Early stage
Begin with B-1, B-2, B-19, B-28 & C-40

Rehabilitation Late stage
Progress to B-1, B-27 & B-31

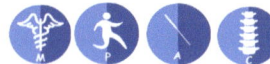

Arm

Arthritis of the shoulder is a chronic degenerative condition. It is most commonly a result of excessive use of the joint and improper joint mechanics (bad working posture, slouching, weak back muscles). The cardinal signs of arthritis in the shoulder are a slow progressive onset of pain (years), a dull and achy character of pain and reduced range of motion. Having a history of shoulder injuries and shoulder pain that worsens with weather changes are also quite typical of arthritic shoulders.

The crucial first step of management is a proper diagnosis. The typical journey will include a visit to your family doctor, X-rays, and then referral to a physiotherapist. Chiropractors and Osteopaths are a good first choice as well. Your doctor will take X-rays to confirm or rule out joint degeneration. Your examination should include a thorough physical exam as well. In brief, your best options are rehabilitation, strengthening programs and a variety of conservative therapies. It is important to understand that your body adapts to the demands placed on it. A chronic degenerative condition like osteoarthritis in the shoulder is a sign that the demands on that joint have been imbalanced for a long time. Rehabilitating a shoulder is the process of changing the way you use the arm so that using it becomes productive instead of destructive. A helpful piece of advice is to exercise a lot and remain active. It is unproductive to avoid activities and nurse your arm too much.

Avoid ballistic activities, heavy lifting and activities that cause pain. Activities like swimming, golf, bowling, yoga, stretching and light resistance training are all encouraged as long as they are tolerated well.

It is *very* important for those with problematic shoulders to develop and maintain proper upper back and shoulder postures. See chapter on Optimal Biomechanics.

Cortisone injections are a good option only when symptoms become severe or conservative treatment is unsuccessful. There is little to no therapeutic benefit to an analgesic or cortisone shot, but it offers temporary relief of symptoms, which can sometimes help expedite the recovery process. End of the line surgery typically consists of arthroplasty with a prosthetic implant. If your doctor thinks it's degenerated and problematic enough, you will likely get referred for a consultation with an orthopaedic surgeon.

Therapies that might help include: Acupuncture, mobilizations done by a well-trained practitioner, massage therapy, laser therapy, electrotherapy, hot or cold packs, capsaicin or menthol creams.

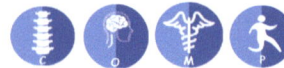

SUGGESTED TREATMENT

SHORT TERM

It has long been known that a strong relation exists between nutrition and arthritis. Arthritis is after all an issue involving inflammation and what we ingest profoundly affects our ability to deal with inflammation. There are a number of nutrients that can have a powerful effect when supplemented. A short list of the most well-supported options are listed at the end of this chapter under Osteoarthritis. Consult a healthcare practitioner, then be patient, results are slow and subtle.

Rehabilitation in the early stages should consist of; B-31, B-28, B-2, B-3, B-8, C-40 and C-41

LONG TERM

Progress into C-43 and C-24

Rehabilitation: Late stage
After 4 weeks with the pictured exercises, begin with D-1, B-14, B-27 & D-6

Perform the following stretches as frequently as possible throughout the week.

B-18

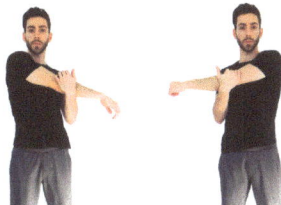

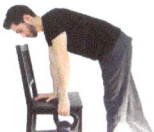

C-4

B-14

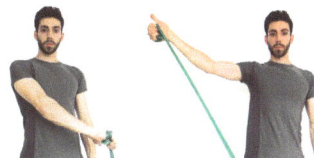

B-30

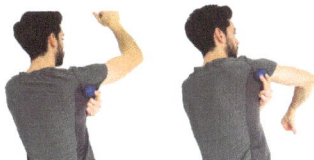

B-30

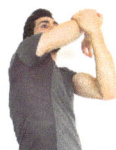

C-41

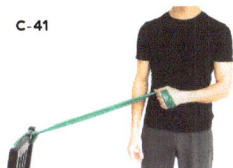

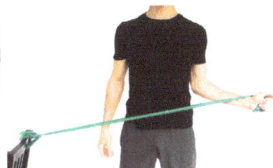

C-40

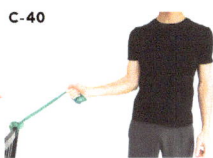

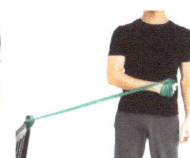

Full descriptions of stretches are in Exercise Appendix

Arm

Thoracic Outlet Syndrome (TOS) is a condition where the structures at the base of the neck tighten and compress the vessels (arteries, veins and nerves) travelling through the area. This causes symptoms into the arms, neck and chest. The typical case of TOS causes numbness, tingling (or pins & needles) into the arms. It can be one arm or both, involves a constant ache from the neck down into the arm and is often accompanied by numbness and tingling along the inside part of the forearm and hand. These types of pains often get worse at night and when doing specific tasks with the arms (like blow drying or lifting the hand above the shoulder).

TOS can also (less commonly) cause constantly cold hands and white fingers, or swollen arms and hands.

Visit your massage therapist and request that they work on your 'scalenes'. Spend as much time as you can stretching. Then strengthening the muscles of the area help correct the imbalances in the long term.

Self-test: while sitting, hold your arms up with your elbows bent and begin making 'quacking' movements with your hands as fast as possible. Start a timer and continue doing this for 3 minutes. If you can do this for 3 minutes without symptoms, then keep investigating for the cause of your symptoms. If symptoms develop within 3 minutes, it is indicative of TOS.

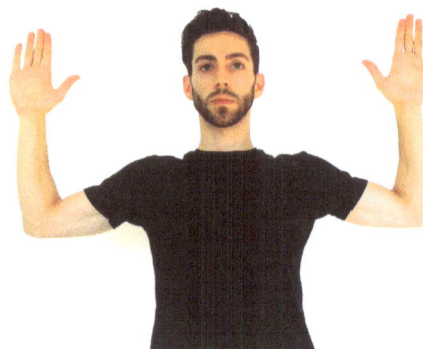

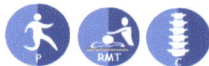

SUGGESTED TREATMENT

SHORT TERM

Perform the following stretches and exercises daily: A-9, A-13, B-5, B-20

Using a posture brace or kinesiology tape while working for 2-3 weeks

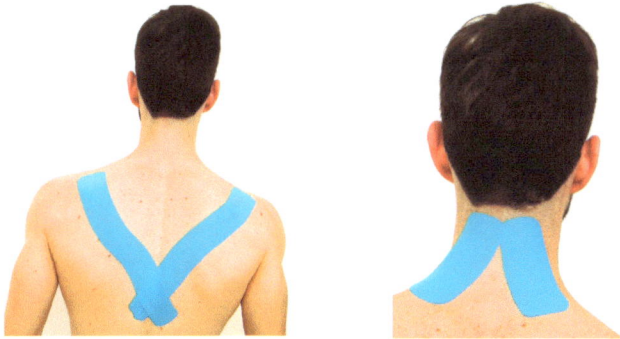

LONG TERM

Perform B-24, B-25, B-29 at least 3 times per week.

Work on improving shoulder blade retraction while working.

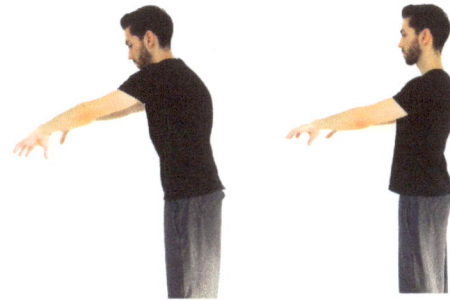

Bad   Good

Rehabilitation: Early stage
Begin with A-5, B-22 & B-32
Rehabilitation: Late stage
Progress to B-1, B-26 & B-27

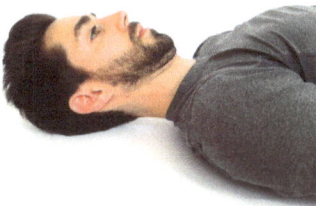

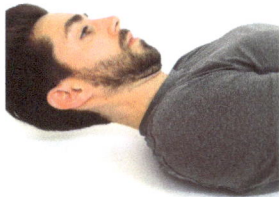

A - 5

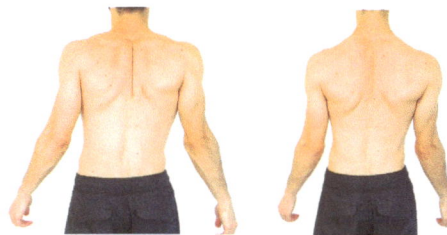

B-32

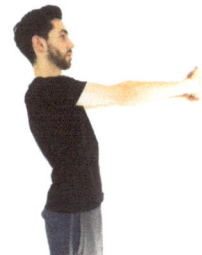

B-22

Neck

If you have a **'kink in your neck'**, sharp pains shoot through your neck when you move into certain positions. This happens when the facet joints between the vertebrae of your neck are stuck slightly out of place and not moving properly. Your first stop should be the chiropractors office. In many cases the kink can be resolved after just one or two treatments.

Managing the issue on your own is best done with plenty of gentle movement. Do NOT wear a neck brace and do NOT be afraid of moving your neck. Use heat packs, warm baths, massage, gentle stretching and make sure to avoid excessive screen time (computers, phone, T.V., etc.).

Reflect on how you slept the night or two before your neck started to hurt and if relevant, change your pillow or sleeping position for the next few nights. It is also important to be mindful of the positions you work and relax in. If you sit on the couch to watch tv with your head tilted to one side, use your shoulder to hold a phone to your ear, have your computer screen slightly to one side, or do anything else with your neck in an obscure position.. then it's likely that you've identified the source of your problem. Change the way you do these things and you'll have a much happier neck.

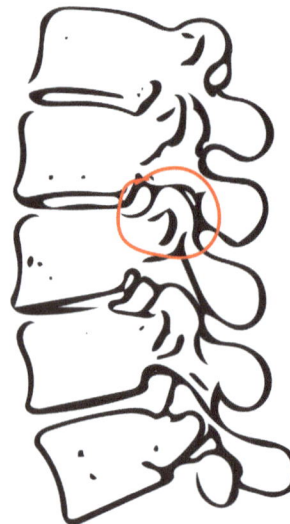

The facet joint between the vertebrae in your neck

94

SUGGESTED TREATMENT

SHORT TERM

Use a neck pillow, heat pack, hot shower or bath, gentle self-massage, topical muscle relaxants (menthol or capsaicin-based, or over-the-counter muscle relaxant cream) and very gentle stretching.

You can do A-2 and A-4 up to several times a day

LONG TERM

Since such joint issues are quick to develop and quick to resolve, the best long term strategy is improving your working postures to prevent further strain. Consult section on Optimal Biomechanics. If your neck problems do not resolve quickly or are recurring frequently, seek a diagnosis from a qualified health professional.

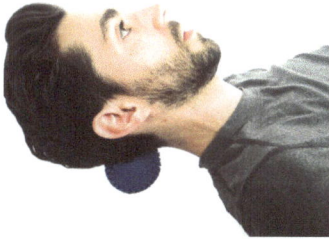

A - 2

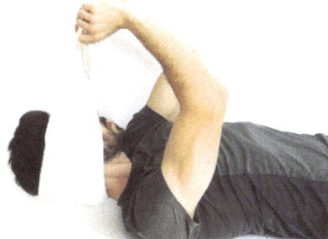

A - 4

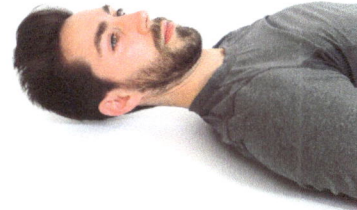

Rehabilitation: Early stage
Begin with A-14
Rehabilitation: Late stage
Progress to A-5 & A-6

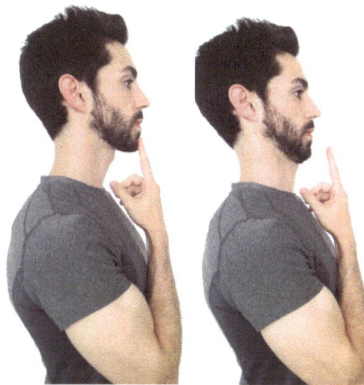

A - 14

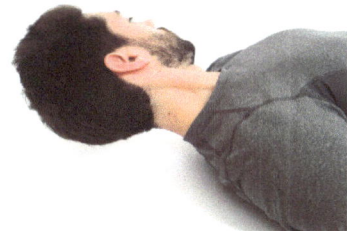

A - 5

Head

Headaches are cumbersome. Most cases of recurring headaches can be resolved, or at least significantly reduced in intensity. Since there are many different types of headaches, each with different causes and contributing factors, our first priority is to figure out which category your headaches fit into.

Note: This chart is meant to be helpful in differentiating between common types of headaches. It does not include considerations of serious medical pathologies, injuries or complications, nor is it meant to substitute for a medical diagnosis. Furthermore, headaches can differ from one person to the next and there may be an overlap in symptoms between types of headaches.

Symptom	Migraine	Tension	Cluster
Intensity, duration & quality of pain			
Mild or moderate pain	✔	✔	
Severe pain	✔		
Lasts 30 min – 7 days		✔	
Lasts 4-72 hours	✔		
Pounding or throbbing and debilitating	✔		✔
Distracting but not debilitating		✔	
Steady ache		✔	
Happen in frequent bouts			✔
Location of pain			
One side of head	✔		✔
Both sides of head	✔	✔	
Behind the eye			✔
Associated Symptoms			
Nausea/vomiting	✔		
Sensitivity to light or sound	✔		
Auro comes on before headache	✔		
Nasal congestion, runny nose, bothered eyes			✔

Head

Migraines are nasty creatures, as anyone who has ever had one can attest to. While we don't know precisely what causes them, most theories purport that migraines are a neurological issue and that symptoms are predominantly caused by changes in the blood flow to the head. They are mostly triggered by hormonal changes, chemical triggers or irregular neurological activity in the brain. Triggers can be emotional - caused by a mental state (like stress), foods or substances, medications, or shifts in levels of certain hormones or sugar in the blood. Rarely, migraines can be caused by underlying medical issues. It is therefore important for regular migraine sufferers to be screened by their family physician. Blood tests, neurological exams and blood pressure assessments can help to rule out potential causes or contributing factors. Typically however, there is no obvious underlying medical problem, and migraine sufferers are left to learn how to manage their condition on their own.[17]

The typical migraine develops in four stages: prodrome, aura, headache and postdrome. The prodrome can consist of fatigue, constipation, muscle stiffness, diarrhea, mood changes, drowsiness or yawning for hours or even days before a migraine attack. The aura stage presents variable sensory phenomena that lasts an hour or less and can include visual disturbances (halo vision or flashing lights), numbness or hypersensitivity in limbs, smelling imaginary odors, vertigo or auditory hallucinations. The headache phase is generally the most unbearable part of a migraine episode. Symptoms can include pain - worsened by physical activity, nausea, vomiting, diarrhea or constipation, nasal congestion, anxiety, hot flashes, chills, dizziness, dehydration or fluid retention, sensitivity to light and sensitivity to sound. If symptoms ever last for longer than 72 hours you should seek medical attention.

Below is a list of common dietary triggers.[18] Monitor your intake of these substances and keep track of the ones that correspond to migraine episodes.

Phenylethylamine - a component of cocoa (chocolate). It causes the release of chemicals that increase the activity of blood vessels in the brain.

Tyramine - found in aged cheese, cured meats, smoked fish, beer, fermented food and yeast extract among other things. It stimulates the sympathetic nervous system.

Aspartame - the popular artificial sweetener. It has numerous other detrimental health effects too, you're best off just avoiding the stuff.

MSG - the flavour enhancer widely used in Asian Cuisine and canned/processed food. It causes unnatural constriction or dilation of blood vessels, particularly at high doses.

Nitrates/Nitrites - preservatives that are used to colour food, lengthen shelf life or add a smoked flavour. They cause a release of nitric oxide and cause blood vessels to dilate.

Alcohol - particularly red wine is a trigger for many migraine sufferers. Wine contains tyramine, sulfites, histamine and phenolic flavonoids, all of which can be troublesome.

Caffeine - comes in (relatively) natural forms, in coffees and teas and dark chocolate. It also comes in many non-natural forms, like energy drinks. Ironically it can also be found in many prescription headache medications. Caffeine causes the blood vessels in the brain to constrict and releases excitatory neurotransmitters.

Head

Some migraine sufferers (about 20%) will experience an aura or prodrome, which are symptoms that proceed the onset of the migraine by an hour or two. It can be sensitivity to light or smell, visual disturbances or other neurological disturbances.

Managing migraines is best done by making several efforts simultaneously.

•Identify and control triggers. Keep a journal to monitor diet, exposure to chemicals and toxins, menstrual cycle and stress levels. Watch for patterns and relate them temporally to the onset of your headaches.

•Stress control. Seek out a method of stress relief that you will enjoy. It can be meditation, exercise, yoga, a therapist or many other things. Just be consistent.

•Trigger point therapy. Have a massage therapist work on your head and neck.

•Biofeedback relaxation therapy. It can help you have more influence over activity of your nervous system, helping you to reduce chronic stress.

•Acupuncture. There are specific acupuncture protocols that can be effective for migraines.

•Nutrition. Avoid food triggers, do not skip meals, and make an effort to improve your general diet. Some sources suggest that the following are useful to supplement: Feverfew, 5-HTP (5-hydroxy-tryptophan), omega-3 oils, calcium, vitamin D,

riboflavinoids, magnesium, vitamin B2 & B6.[19]

•Pharmaceuticals. Ask your MD about certain prescription medications can help. I don't recommend this as the first course of action because it usually delays the efforts you would otherwise make towards treating the cause.

•Sleep. Improving the quality of your sleep can have positively effects for migraine sufferers. Ensure to sleep in a fully dark room and avoid under or over sleeping. See chapter on Sleep.

•Intravenous IV vitamin C therapy can be an effective treatment in some cases, for both migraines and for general pain syndromes.

•Botox injections have been used effectively to relieve pain in the TMJ (the jaw) and the neck, which can improve the state of migraines.

The following is a list of herbs and supplements that can help prevent or treat migraines.[20] The list descends in order of the quality of evidence that supports it. Consult a physician before taking a new supplement.
Magnesium (400mg daily)
Petasites hybridus (Butterbur) (75mg twice daily for 1 month, then 50mg twice daily)
Feverfew (100mg daily)
CoQ10 (300mg daily)
Riboflavin/B2 (400mg daily)
Alpha lipoid acid (600mg daily)

Head

(Cervicogenic) tension headaches

Cervicogenic means 'from the cervical spine' (the neck). A cervicogenic tension headache is most commonly caused by tension in the neck muscles. When you have such a headache it is not always obvious that it's being caused by muscles, but it's certainly worth finding out because it's very treatable (and preventable). This type of tension headache is the kind of headache that comes on when you are overworked and stressed. They tend to begin in the back of the neck or base of the skull and send pain and bands of tension up into the rest of your head. The tight muscles in the neck constrict the blood vessels supplying your head and scalp (worsening the headache).

Stretching several times throughout the day will help to reduce muscle tension; A-1, A-2, A-8, A-9. Heat, massage and topical muscle relaxants will also be very helpful. Long-term management should entail working to improve neck range of motion (keep stretching, add in A-13 and A-11) and reducing forward head posture with A-5 exercise.

Chiropractic adjustments to the neck have been shown to be effective in treating cervicogenic headaches.[21]

Cluster headaches are a type of headache that tends to be severe, recurrent, on one side of the head and most often behind the eye. They are often accompanied by nasal congestion or eye watering. Cluster headaches are difficult to treat, but there are a number of helpful remedies.

Supplementing melatonin (10mg once a day, taken at night) has been shown to be helpful. St. John's Wort can help improve sleep and reduce depression that may accompany chronic headaches. Cluster headache sufferers are often deficient in magnesium and supplementation can help. Capsaicin (the active ingredient in hot peppers) has been shown to reduce the frequency of cluster headaches (though not intensity or symptoms), but only in the form of intranasal civamide treatment (a nasal flush with capsaicin's twin substance).[22] Biofeedback therapy has also been shown to help reduce cluster headaches.[23]

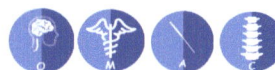

Note: Headaches are sometimes associated strongly with your emotions just as they are with your physical condition. They have been consistently linked to levels of sleep, energy and levels of social engagement. Frustration, anger, fear, anxiety and depression will all contribute to headaches. In you're efforts to relieve the discomfort of headaches, don't neglect the importance of addressing any emotional struggles.

Upper Back

General upper back soreness (Cervicothoracic postural strain)

I would be surprised if you don't have frequent soreness in your upper back; most hairstylists do. As do people who work at desks, have poor posture, sit too often, work with their hands, and even those who get stressed out easily. I generally recommend that people manage this problem both passively and actively. Passive solutions may include massage, chiropractic, acupuncture, etc. Active solutions are activities that improve your postural strength and flexibility - yoga, Pilates, stretching, lifting weights, etc. The best approach is to combine your favorite bits of both types of solutions. I recommend visiting your chiropractor, massage therapist, osteopath or acupuncturist a few times consecutively to give yourself a head-start on this journey towards a strong and relaxed upper back. The rest of the journey towards sustaining a happy body is in your hands.

The stretches on the next page will contribute to resolving the tension built up in the muscles of the area. The rehabilitation exercises will help strengthen your postural muscles. The quality of movement is very important while training these muscles, so remember to practice slow smooth movement.

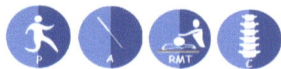

It is useful for some to try a postural support device or postural tape. A simple elastic support system can hold your upper back and shoulders in an improved position. Examples can be found in the 'Helpful Tools' section. Improvements you make to your general and to your working postures will lessen the burden on the tissues of your upper back and will reduce soreness.

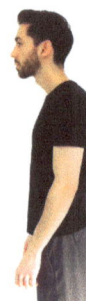
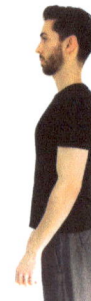

Bad   **Good**

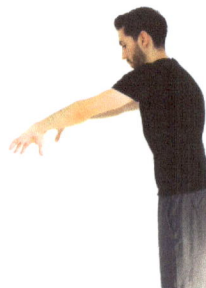
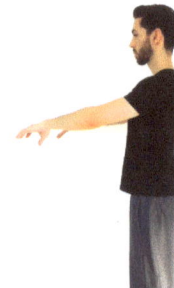

Bad   **Good**

SUGGESTED TREATMENT

SHORT TERM

There are several great stretches and self-treatments that will help resolve your upper back tension. Try them all and choose your 3 favorite to do regularly.

A-1, D-4, A-9, B-4, B-10, B-11, B-21, B-24, B-29, D-2

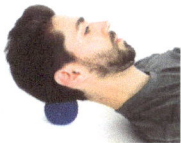
A - 1

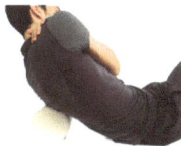
D - 4

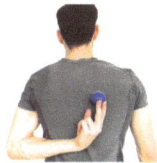
B - 29

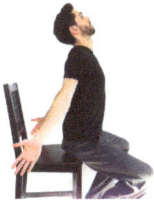
D - 2

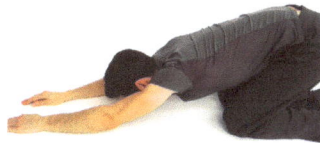
B - 24

LONG TERM

A-25, B-5, A-10, B-9, B-22, B-32, D-3, D-5

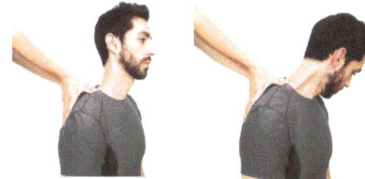
B - 9

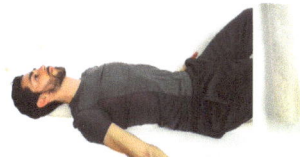
D - 3

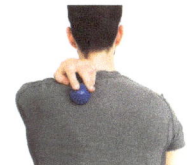
D - 5

Rehabilitation: Early stage
Begin with B-2, B-26, B-27 & H-9

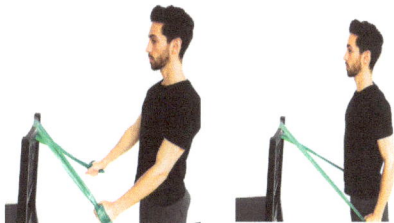
B - 27

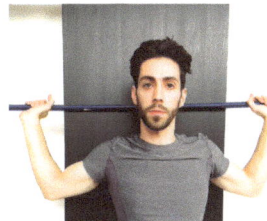
B - 26

Rehabilitation: Late stage
Progress to A-5, B-28 & H-9

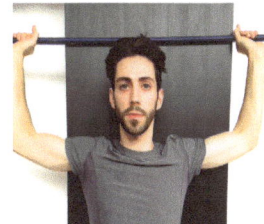

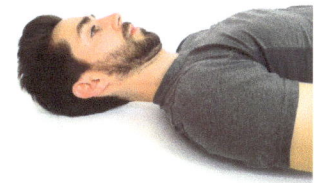
A - 5

Upper Back

Rib that's 'out' (Costovertebral joint subluxation)

One of the more pestering issues to have, the ribs can sometimes shift out of their happy place (neutral position) and put pressure against the capsule that covers them. It can happen as the result of an injury to your rib cage, or it can just happen spontaneously. Unfortunately once aggravated, it can sometimes take a while to settle back down.

When aggravated, it's important to get into a safe position when coughing sneezing or bearing down. Do this by straightening your back and rolling your shoulders back, then avoiding bending forward or twisting. An irritated costovertebral joint is much more common in people with poor posture. Identify the times you spend slumping forward (on the couch, in the car, in an office chair, at work, etc.) and modify your posture. The easiest way is to use a lot of lumbar support to keep your spine upright. For instance, you could roll up a sweater and place it behind your low back the next time you sit on the couch or in a car.

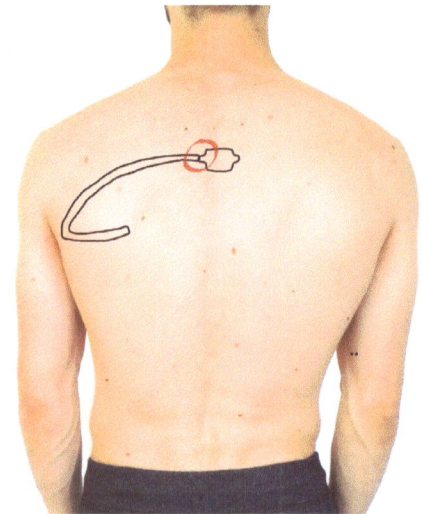

A costovertebral joint - the joint where the rib meets the vertebrae

SUGGESTED TREATMENT

SHORT TERM

Consider a short-term kinesiology tape application to help protect the rib movement. Use D-3, B-6 and B-25 to help reduce the strain on the area.

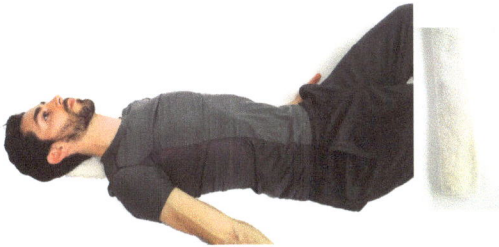

D - 3

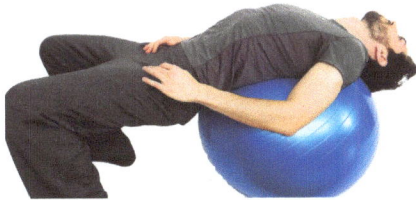

B - 25

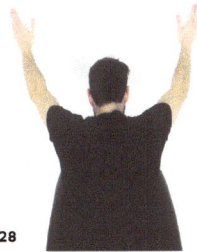

B - 28

Rehabilitation: Early stage
Begin with B-28 & B-22
Rehabilitation: Late stage
Progress to B-1, B-7 & D-1

LONG TERM

Continue with D-2, B-29 and consider the use of a postural brace for a few weeks while you strengthen the torso muscles.

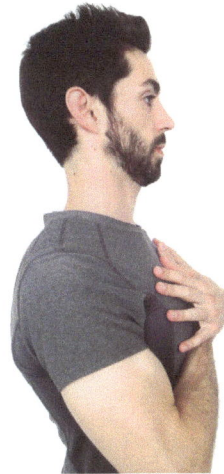

Rib cage reset
Cross your arms over your chest, stand up straight & tall, tuck your chin in, roll your shoulders back. Now take 10 slow deep breaths, focusing on lifting your diaphragm and expanding your chest forward.

Upper Back

Sternum pains (Costosternal syndrome/Costochondritis)

When it comes to chest pain, we must be cautious. Anytime someone experiences symptoms like tightness or sharp pains in the chest it is most important to rule out issues involving the heart and lungs. In the case of costosternal syndrome, there is one crucial factor that leads us to suspect that the problem is caused by irritation of the sternal joints and not something more serious: if the pain is *completely* reproducible by pushing on a specific point on the sternum or one of the ribs, then we can assume that we are dealing with a cartilage or capsule issue. That said, always see a medical professional immediately if you are having chest pains of any kind.

This condition most often occurs after an injury, a severe bout of coughing, aggressive exercise (most often pectoral workouts), or as a result of chronically bad postural habits. It is more common in women. It presents as sharp shooting pains in the sternum area, usually on one side, and is aggravated by pushing on the spot, by coughing, sneezing and vigorous torso movements.

Dealing with it involves first avoiding aggravating activities. Break up the amount to time you spend in forward bending or hunched positions. Get up to do a quick stretch for every 20 minutes you spend sitting down or reaching forwards. Make sure to spend time in the position shown in D-3 every day. If it is painful to stretch, see a therapist first.

Work out the tension in the muscles that pull on the area (mostly the pectoralis major) by stretching and rolling on a ball.

Remember that each rib has joints in the front of your chest as well as in the back along your vertebrae. That implies value in spending time improving the condition of the sets of ribs and the muscles throughout your midback. See the section on 'Sore Upper Back' for suggestions.

Finally, you'll want to improve your posture to prevent this from recurring. A-5, B-1 and B-27 will get you on your way.

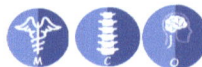

SUGGESTED TREATMENT

SHORT TERM

When dealing with an acutely irritated rib, the best things to do are rest, alternate ice and heat, take cough suppressants or anti-inflammatories if needed, and begin gently stretching the pectorals (B-5, B-6). Use D-3 to relax the whole ribcage.

LONG TERM

If your symptoms do not improve, then seek a follow up medical consultation. Chiropractic or osteopathic adjustments and laser therapy can be helpful.

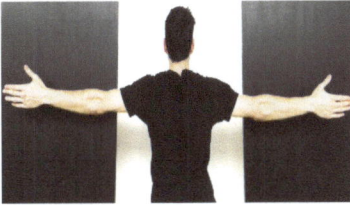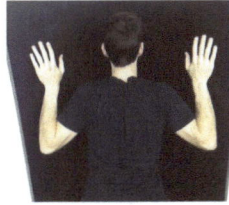

B - 5   B - 6

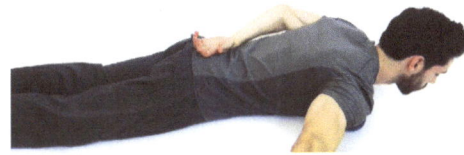

C - 45

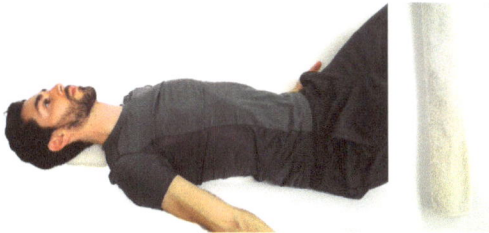

D - 3

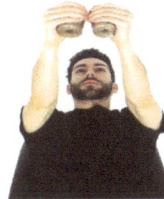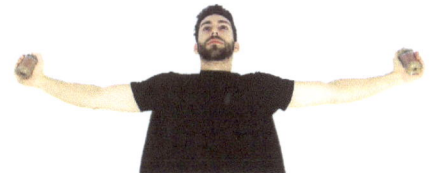

C - 46

Rehabilitation: Early stage
Begin with C-45
Rehabilitation: Late stage
Progress to C-46

Lower Back

Sharp jolts of pain in the low back when bending backwards may be indicative of **facet joint irritation**. Roughly 15-40% of low back pain originates from the facet joints.

When these joints are irritated, you may also experience general back soreness, pain moving into certain positions or pain shooting up or down your back.

The pain comes from the capsule that surrounds the joint. The cause is often multifactorial. Facet joints can shift out of their 'happy position' as a result of excessive sitting, poor form during a workout, leaning to one side too often, wearing high heels too often, repetitive lifting and other forms of muscular imbalances or poor movement habits.

Resolving the pain therefore requires relaxing the aggravated tissues, flexibility work and overall strengthening to prevent recurrence. A visit to your chiropractor may give you some immediate relief and help your body resolve the issue quickly. By adjusting the joints of your spine, the treatment will 'reset' them and will sometimes be all you need. To prevent recurrence, it will be important to increase the diversity of movement in your low back when at work. This means stretching frequently and learning to move/roll your pelvis while standing.

Successful prevention of further episodes requires some investment. Strengthening the muscles that stabilize the movements of the low back is the key to preventing facet irritation (and to a healthy back in general). Long-term prevention is best accomplished with the specific 'big 3' exercises - H-2, H-5 and H-7 in the Exercise Appendix. They are based on the work of Dr. Stuart McGill, a global expert on spinal stability.

SUGGESTED TREATMENT

SHORT TERM

Rest and ice if pain is severe. Once symptoms subside to moderate levels use heat instead of ice.

E-1, F-21, E-2, E-11, H-6

LONG TERM

E-3, E-10, F-23

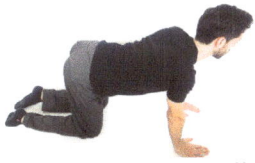
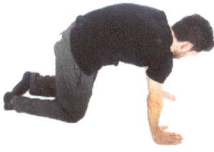

H - 6

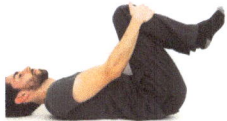

E - 1

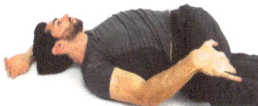

E - 2

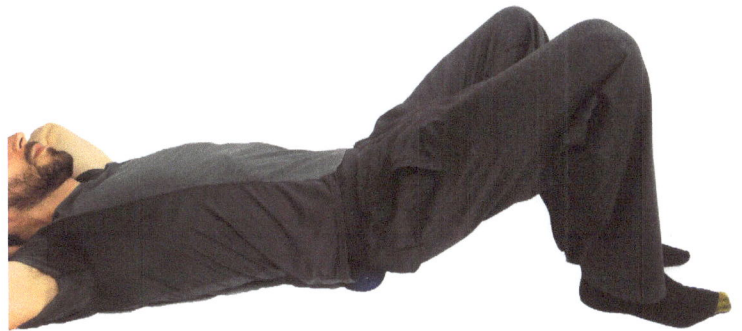

E - 10

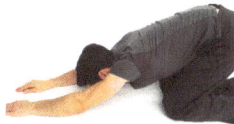

E - 11

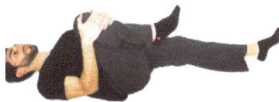

F - 21

Rehabilitation: Early stage
Begin with E-5, H-1 & H-10
Rehabilitation: Late stage
Progress to E-9, H-2, H-3, H-4, H-5 & H-10

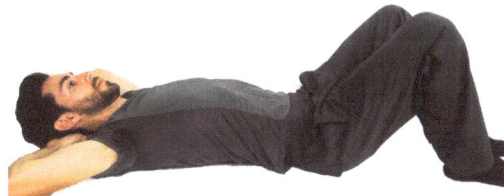

E - 5

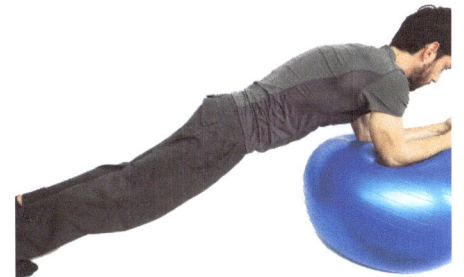

H - 5

Lower Back

Low back sprains/strains are quite tricky. Low back pain is almost always more complicated than a simple muscle strain. The biomechanics of the low back are such that injuries often involve several tissues or start with one problem and snowball into a worse one. That said, I believe the best approach is to use a blanket approach and try to rule in other more specific conditions to ascertain more helpful guidance.

Rest time is only necessary as long as the severity of the pain prevents reasonable movements (usually no more than half of a day). One of the most universally useful positions of relief is lying on your back with your knees bent to 90 degrees and your legs supported (by a pillow/chair/couch etc.).

After the initial bout of pain begins to settle, think MOVEMENT. You may be timid about getting up and moving around, but know that it is almost always more therapeutic than resting. Just keep your activities moderate and take plenty of breaks.

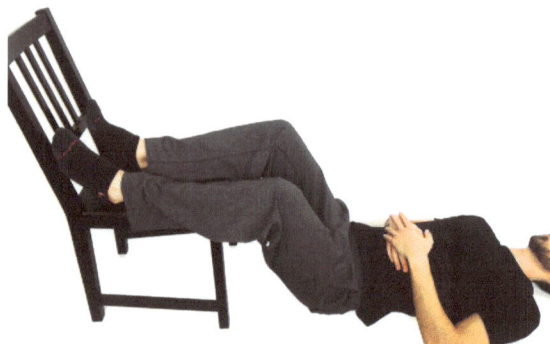

SUGGESTED TREATMENT

SHORT TERM

If you're not up to walking around or doing yoga, spend as much time as you can using F-20 and H-6 to reduce the pain and quicken your recovery.

LONG TERM

E-2 (with knees bent), E-7, E-8, F-12

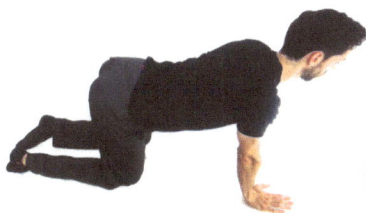 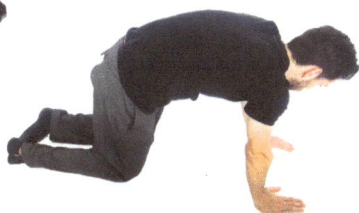

H - 6

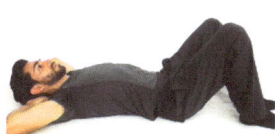

E - 8

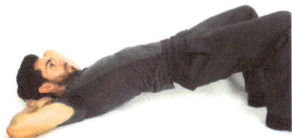 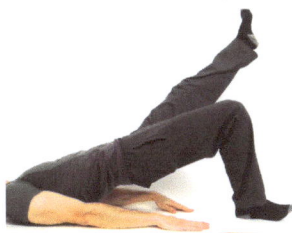

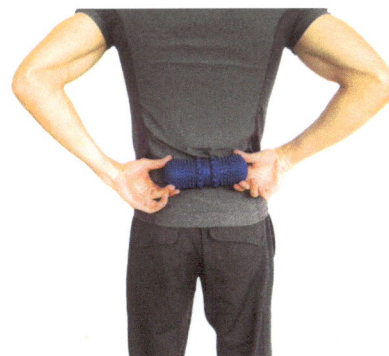

E - 7

Rehabilitation: Early stage
Begin with H-1, F-10, F-11 & F-12
Rehabilitation: Late stage
Progress to H-1, H-2, H-3, H-4, H-5, H-7, F-14, F-18, F-19, F-13, F-8 & E-18

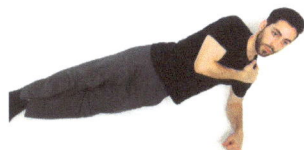

H - 3

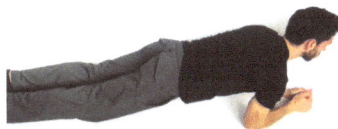

H - 4

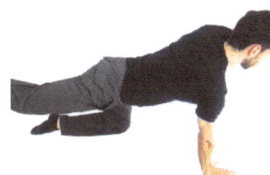 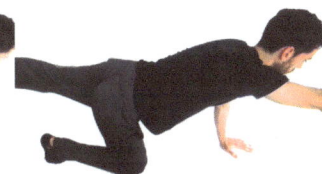

H - 7

Lower Back

A **sacroiliac joint sprain** can be differentiated from low back issues by noting a slightly lower point of pain. The Sacroiliac (SI) joints are the two joints formed where the tailbone meets the pelvis. The joints are held together by strong thick ligaments and are not meant to move much. Too much or too little movement can cause problems and lead to pain. When an SI joint is sprained, bending at the hips is usually very painful. Most movements that hinge at the pelvis will be particularly aggravating, like getting up from a sitting position, getting out of a car, bending backwards or shifting your weight from one leg to the other.

The joints change during pregnancy, which can become problematic. SI pain can sometimes be hard to identify. SI pain tends to manifest in the area depicted in blue. The task of distiguishing it from lower back problems should be left to a professional.

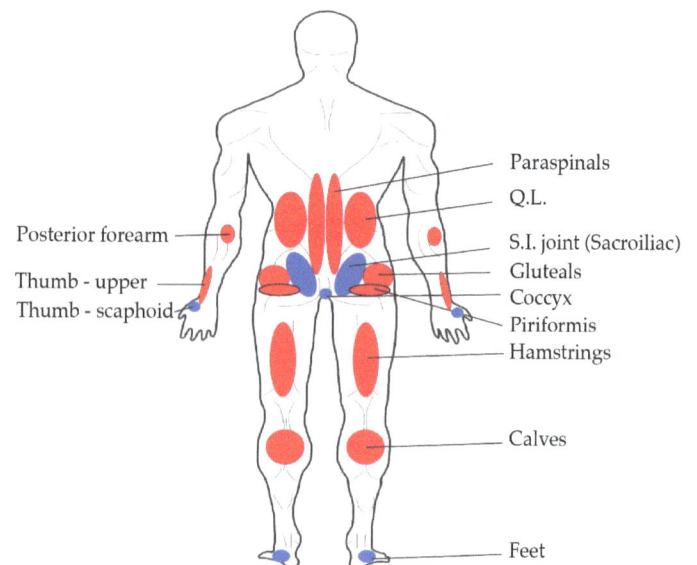

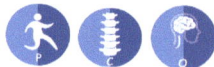

Posterior forearm
Thumb - upper
Thumb - scaphoid

Paraspinals
Q.L.
S.I. joint (Sacroiliac)
Gluteals
Coccyx
Piriformis
Hamstrings

Calves

Feet

SUGGESTED TREATMENT

SHORT TERM

To help with an irritated SI joint, we want to relax the tight muscles in the area, work toward re-aligning the pelvic and sacral bones and then work on improving the coordination of the muscles in the area.

For really intense bouts of pain, I recommend using a 'SI Belt' for several days. It will help to minimize movement of the SI joints and reduce pain.

Start with E-13, E-14, F-21, H-6 and E-15

LONG TERM

E-2, F-23, E-8, E-3, E-10

Learn to avoid leaning more on one leg than the other.

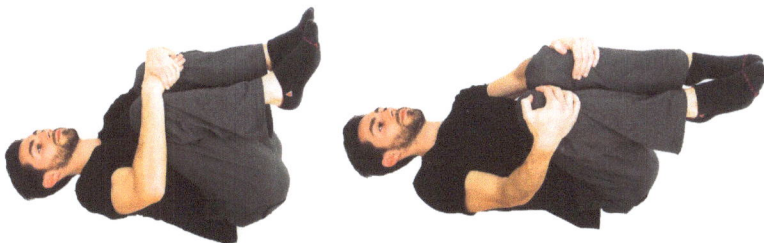

E - 14

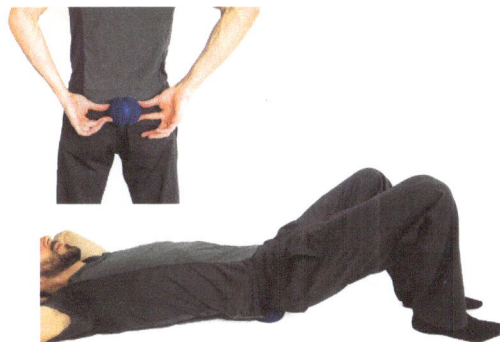

E - 13

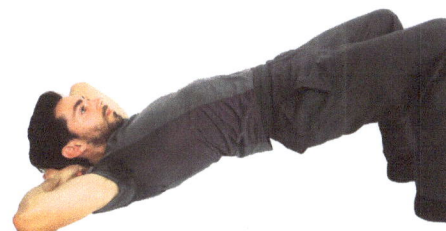

E - 15

Rehabilitation: Early stage
Begin with H-7, H-1, F-18, F-19, F-24 or F-25
Rehabilitation: Late stage
Progress to H-2, H-3, H-4, H-5, E-16, E-17 & E-18

Lower Back

Piriformis syndrome is a condition in which the piriformis muscle tightens and compresses the sciatic nerve causing pain in the buttocks and down the leg. A good number of people suffering from 'sciatica' are experiencing the effects of piriformis syndrome.

It most often plagues people with distinct muscle imbalances, differences in leg length and those who sit too much. The piriformis muscles are responsible for rotating the hips outwards. They can be strained and overworked when the muscles of the pelvis and hips are not balanced or strong enough. The other common cause of pain radiating down the leg is a disc herniation, which is a more severe injury, often beginning immediately (as opposed to developing progressively) and accompanied by debilitating pain. Piriformis syndrome tends to come and go, develop over time and is provoked when your heel first hits the ground while you walk.

Managing it is a matter of first reducing tension in the muscle, then bringing balance back to the pelvis and hips.

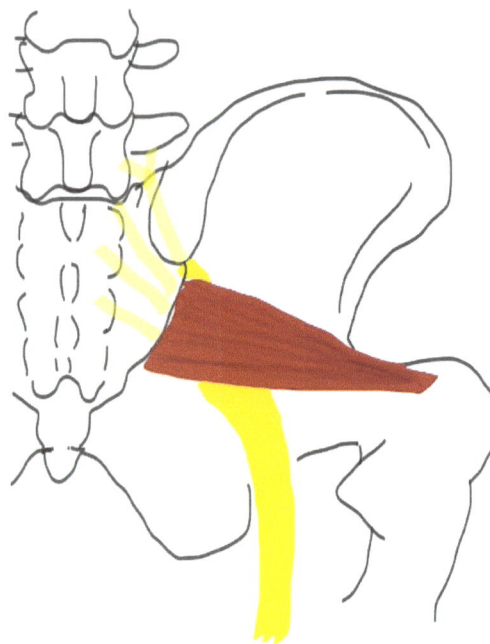

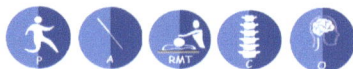

SUGGESTED TREATMENT

SHORT TERM

The short term goal is to stretch the piriformis and the surrounding tissues gently to help it all relax. Use F-7, F-8, F-21 and F-31.

LONG TERM

The longer term goal is to improve overall hip movements. Use F-22, F-23, F-10 and F-30.

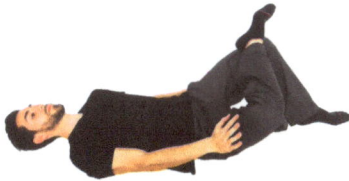

F - 8

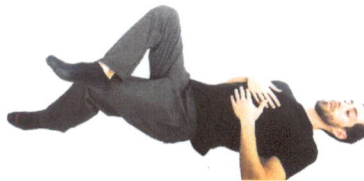

F - 7

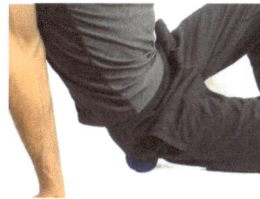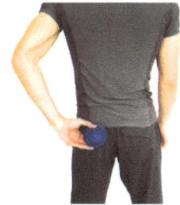

F - 22

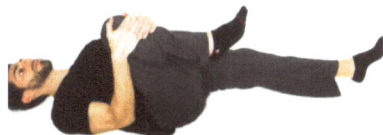

F - 21

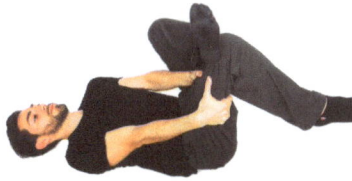

F - 31

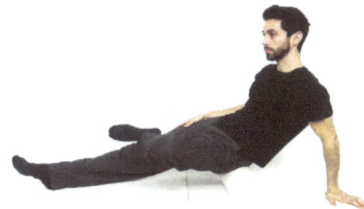

F - 23

Rehabilitation: Early stage
Begin with F-30 & H-8
Rehabilitation: Late stage
Progress to F-18 & F-19

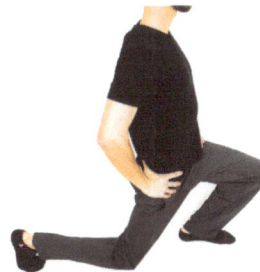

F - 10

Lower Back

Trochanteric bursitis is an inflammation of the large bursa on the outermost point of the hip. A bursa is a fluid filled sac that provides cushioning to bony parts of your body. Trochanteric bursitis is easily identified by sharp or intense pain upon pushing (even lightly) on the bony prominence on either hip.

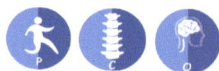

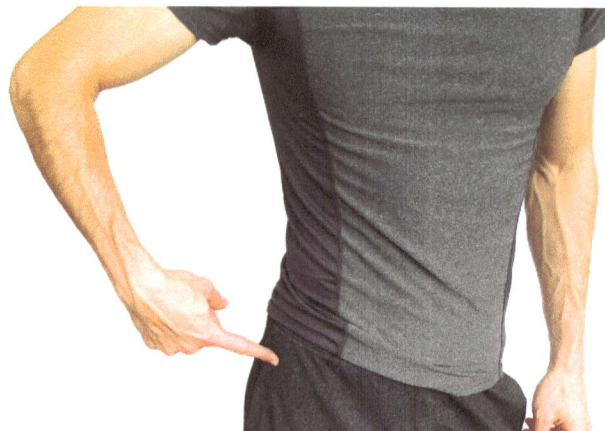

SUGGESTED TREATMENT

SHORT TERM

Ice, rest, avoid prolonged sitting, E-1, F-12,

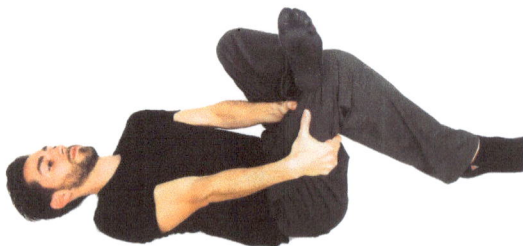

F - 12

LONG TERM

Use F-29 to reduce tension in the gluteus medius.

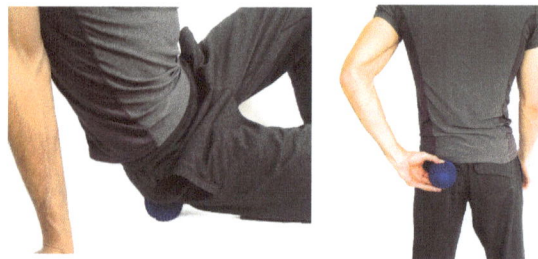

F - 29

Lower Back

Hip joint pain

The hips are incredibly tough and resilient joints. When considering hip pain, it's important not to neglect any symptoms or subtle issues. Not only does it take quite a bit of strain to cause hip pain but when the hips are not working optimally, the rest of your body suffers from the resulting asymmetries in you movement. Improper hip movements (even minor changes) can very quickly cause back pain/strain, knee, ankle and foot problems.

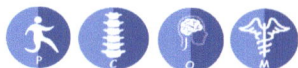

SUGGESTED TREATMENT

SHORT TERM

F-8, F-10, F-11, F-27, F-29, F-21 and F-30

LONG TERM

F-11, F-16 and E-8

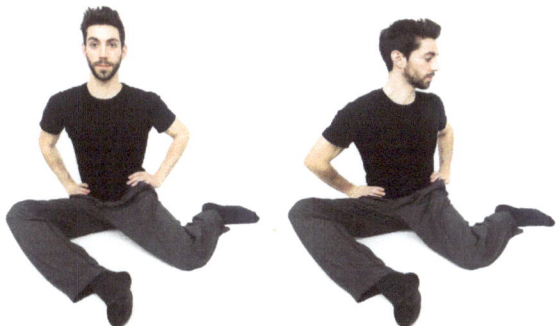

F - 30

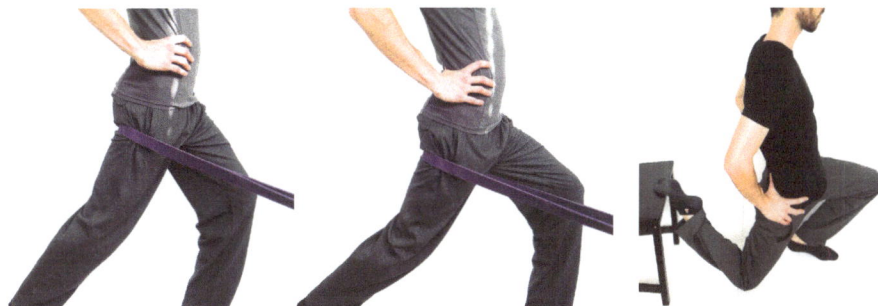

F - 27   F - 11

Rehabilitation: Early stage

Begin with F-27 & H-11

Rehabilitation: Late stage

Progress to F-25, F-18, F-19 & H-14

Legs

Plantar Fasciitis is a painful condition on the bottom of the foot that more commonly afflicts people who stand all day. If the first few steps you take in the morning are excruciatingly painful and have tenderness along the length of the underside of your foot, you may have plantar fasciitis. It is a condition where the tight band of tendon underneath your foot starts to get stretched and damaged, making it very painful to put a lot of weight on the foot. The initial stretching of the tendon could be caused by a variety of things, but often it is the result of walking or running in poor footwear. This causes tearing in the tendon tissue, and as you rest it overnight, your body tries to heal it by laying down scar tissue. This scar tissue protectively pulls the tendon tight and shortens it. When you wake up and take your first step it rapidly stretches, causing micro-tears in the tissue.

The daily tearing and repairing that happens is a cycle that makes it a difficult condition to resolve. A bout of plantar fasciitis can last several months. Once the cycle is broken, it does not take long for the pain to completely disappear.

To effectively reduce the symptoms of plantar fasciitis, you will need to address the cause (throw away those bad shoes, work to correct asymmetries between your two legs, etc.) and you'll need to break the cycle of repeated daily injury. Breaking the cycle can sometimes be as simple as altering your normal daily activities and wearing a night brace/tension sock at night (see helpful tools section). Other helpful remedies include extensive stretching of the feet and calves, specific tape jobs, getting a padded insole for your shoes, having a manual therapist perform cross-friction massage or shockwave therapy ™. Ultrasound therapy is popular but has not been consistently shown to be effective.

Taping your foot as shown below will help reduce the tension on the fascia in most cases. Although it's ideal to have a therapist apply the tape for you, you can do it yourself. Remove immediately if pains begin anywhere else in your foot. Use the tape for a few days, if no problems arise and it seems to help, continue to use it up to a maximum of 3 weeks.

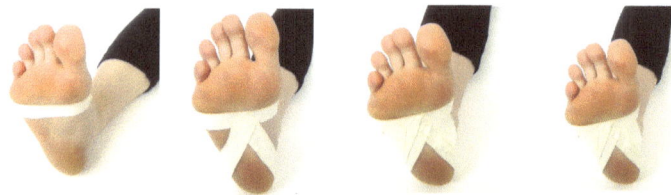

Try wearing a plantar fasciitis night brace for a minimum of 1 week. They can be uncomfortable, but they can be just what you need to break the cycle of repetitive injury.

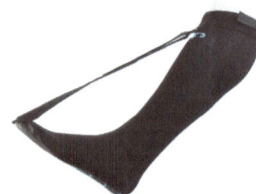

SUGGESTED TREATMENT

SHORT TERM

Rest your foot as much as possible, wear the most supportive footwear you own ALL THE TIME for several days, avoid being barefoot, wear a plantar fasciitis night splint, try a tape job (previous page), roll your foot on a bottle of frozen water and do G-1, G-2, G-3 and G-4 daily.

LONG TERM

If it persists, you'll want to work to improve the condition of the rest of the foot to make sure you are addressing all potentially related issues. Use G-5 and G-11. Spend time on a wobble board and don't forget the G-6 rehabilitation exercise.

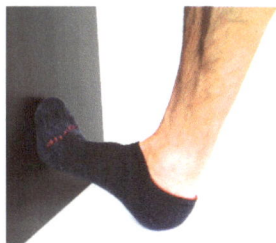

G - 1

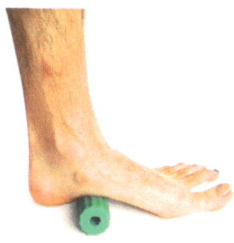

G - 2

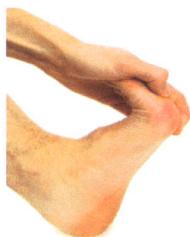

G - 3

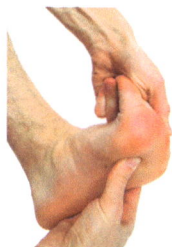

G - 4

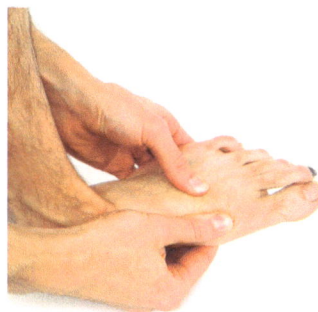

G - 5

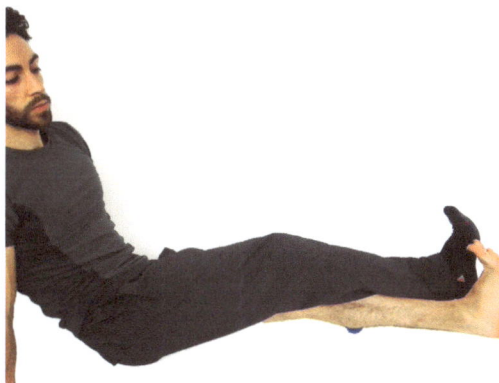

D - 11

Rehabilitation: Early stage
Begin with G-9, G-10 & G-12
Rehabilitation: Late stage
Progress to G-6 & G-8

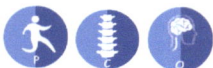

Legs

Sore feet can be the result of a variety of factors, but the most significant factor is certainly footwear. Since you stand for the vast majority of your time working, your shoes must be more supportive than the standard shoe. I'm not suggesting Birkenstocks, but I do think most stylists need to put a little extra thought and preparation into their shoe purchases. It is very possible to find attractive shoes that are also supportive; we just need to make sure they meet a few criteria. Refer to the chapter on Choosing Good Footwear.

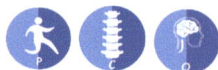

SUGGESTED TREATMENT

SHORT TERM

Re-consider your footwear. Take epsom salt baths in the evening. Incorporate G-2, G-5 and G-17 into your daily routine for a few weeks.

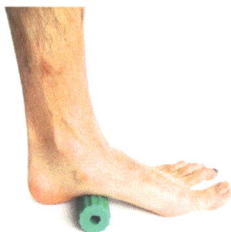 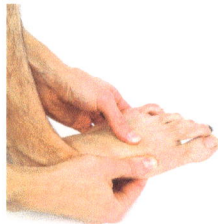

G - 2   G - 5

Rehabilitation: Early stage

G-6

LONG TERM

If your soreness persists, begin working on some of the muscles in the calf that affect the foot. G-16 and G-12

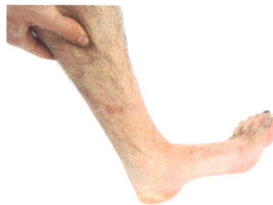 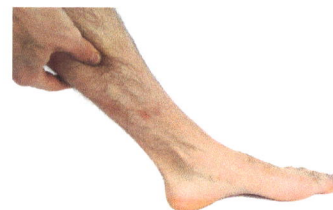

G - 16

Rehabilitation: Late stage

G-7 and G-15

Legs

Big toe pain will often be a combination of sharp stabbing pain and a dull ache. In hairstylists it's typically caused by mechanical strain to the capsule around the big toe joint. It's important to rule out gout or a bunion. Read about bunions on the next page. Gout is very painful condition where uric acid crystals collect in the vessels of the big toe. It happens as a result of a metabolic imbalance or a poor diet. It comes on quite quickly, produces intense sharp pain and often causes the toe to be red and swollen. Gout is a best managed nutritionally and with pharmaceuticals through your medical doctor.

Injuries aside, capsule pain in the big toe is most often caused by tightened calves and hip flexors. When this set of muscles becomes tight and short, the foot lifts off the ground sooner as you walk, bending the toe upwards sooner and causing more forces to move through it. Stretching the calf and psoas on the affected leg for several days will be the most effective remedy.

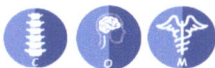

SUGGESTED TREATMENT

SHORT TERM

Reconsider your footwear. Use the following mobilizations consistently; G-2, G-9, G-10, G-12, G-19, G-20 F-10, F-11.

LONG TERM

Consider seing a podiatrist or chiropractor to have custom orthotics made (if the pain hasn't resolved within a 4 weeks). begin doing G-1 and G-5.

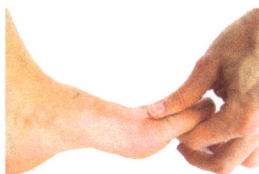

G - 19

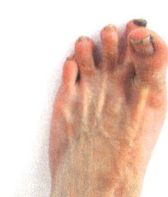

G - 20

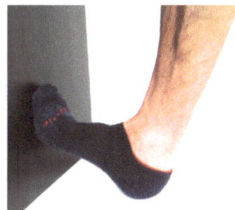

G - 1

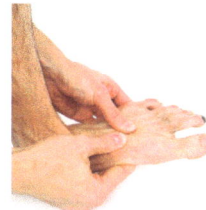

G - 5

Rehabilitation: Early stage

Begin with G-6

Rehabilitation: Late stage

Progress to G-7

Legs

Bunions are every high heel lovers worst nightmare. A bunion is the degeneration and subsequent inward tilting of the first joint of the big toe. It is most often the result of wearing shoes that are too tight around the toes. In a tight or pointy-toed shoe, the big toe is squeezed inwards and the joint (called the first metatarsophalangeal joint) slowly begins to break down and become crooked. The worse they get the more painful (and unattractive) they can become.

Once symptoms are manageable, work up to walking an average of 2 kilometers a day (but not much more) wearing barefoot shoes (Vibram FiveFingers for instance). Ensure you consistently wear shoes with adequate toe space and that don't narrow to a point. As long as you aren't aggravating other joints in the process, barefoot walking can help strengthen the small muscles of the feet that support the toes.

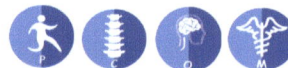

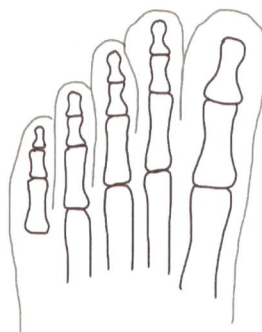

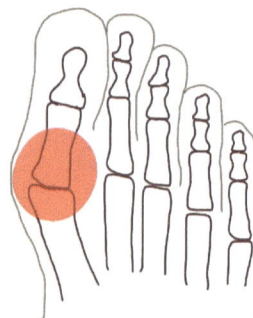

Normal   **Bunion**

SUGGESTED TREATMENT

SHORT TERM

Stop wearing shoes with a narrow or tight toe box. Vary the type of shoes you wear each day as much as possible. Acquire toe-spacers from your drugstore or medical supply center to wear either at night or in your shoes during the day (if possible). To reduce the pain, you may want to bathe your feet in Epsom salts, get a foot massage, and try acupuncture. Consulting a podiatrist, pedorthist or chiropodist is a good idea. Consider a specialized bunion night splint. The tape job shown below is quite effective for mild cases if done consistently for several weeks. G-17 & G-18 are helpful.

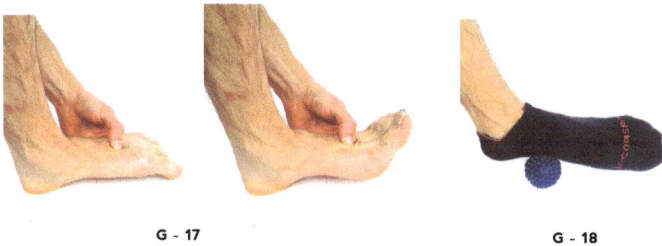

G - 17

G - 18

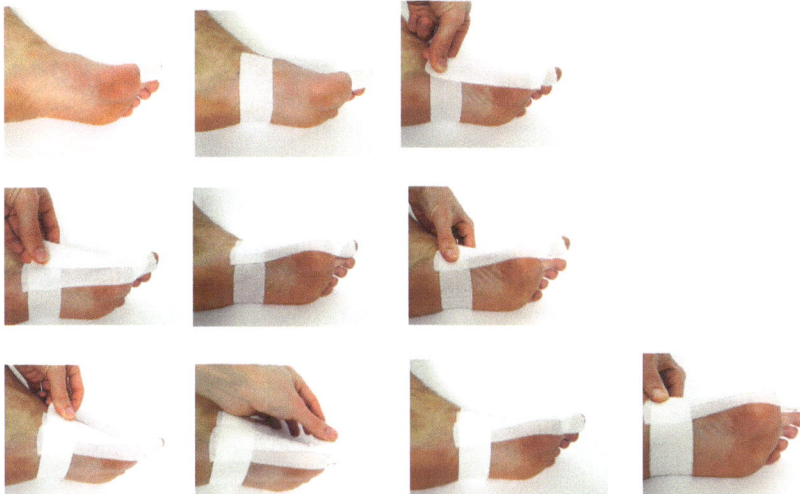

LONG TERM

G-19

Consult with your physician or naturopath about supplementing with glucosamine, chondroitin sulfate, omega-3 & 6 fish oils. They have all been shown to be helpful in improving joint function.[24]

In some more serious cases, certain doctors and specialists can provide steroid injections to reduce pain and swelling in the joint or they may perform surgery. There are several surgical options, the indications for which depend on the case. Recovering from bunion surgery is typically very painful; so take all the warning signs you can to prevent getting to that point.

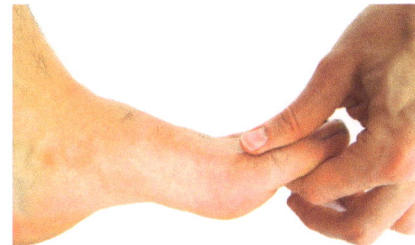

G - 19

Rehabilitation: Early stage
Begin with G-10 & G-20
Rehabilitation: Late stage
Progress to G-15 & G-21

Legs

Sore knees

Knees are able to withstand a lot of compression for long periods of time. This means that standing and walking all day should not cause knee pain or swelling. If you experience sore knees during or after work, there is a problem you need to fix. From my experience the most common knee issues are the result of previous injuries, movement pattern disorders (exacerbated by running or other high caliber activities), and common degeneration (like osteoarthritis). The first step in dealing with knee pain is to get assessed and diagnosed by a professional. Chiropractors, osteopaths, physiotherapists and sports physicians are the best equipped to manage your knee issues. Even if you have sporadic or low level symptoms, I encourage you to seek professional advice. Once you have ruled out specific conditions and causes other than your work, you can consider the various interventions that help ease overall strain on your knees. Wearing well-cushioned shoes or insoles helps to decrease the impact of prolonged weight bearing. Since problems in the foot and ankle can manifest at the knee, ensuring that your footwear is adequately supportive is very helpful.

If you've recently had pain or problems in either of your hips, in your pelvis or low back, keep in mind that it may be related to your knee pain. Make sure to address all related issues.

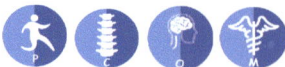

Meniscus damage

The menisci are the two C-shaped pieces of cartilage that are sandwiched between the bones of each knee.

With such a big job, the menisci are quite robust, but can degenerate after decades of wear and tear. They can also get injured during obscure twisting movements, most often during an intense activity. This usually results in a meniscus 'tear'. The way the menisci work is similar to a mortar and pestle. You can imagine that if you had a torn flap of material sticking up from the normally smooth surface of the mortar/bowl, it would 'catch' and get irritated. These injuries are relatively slow to heal and can require surgery if serious enough. While recovering from a meniscus injury, it is important to avoid activities that require twisting of the knees (dancing and most sports).

The first step to managing a meniscus injury is to get diagnosed properly. Once assessed and diagnosed you should first endeavor to heal naturally and rehabilitate before opting for surgery.

Self-treating a meniscus injury is best done with the same protocols as for sore knees, with a heavy focus on the rehabilitation exercises.

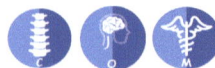

SUGGESTED TREATMENT

SHORT TERM

With knee issues, it is valuable to pay attention to the hip function and to reconsider footwear. Taping the knee can help in the short term. Do G-13 and F-26 daily.

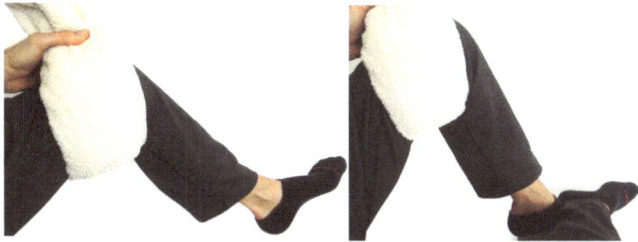

G - 13

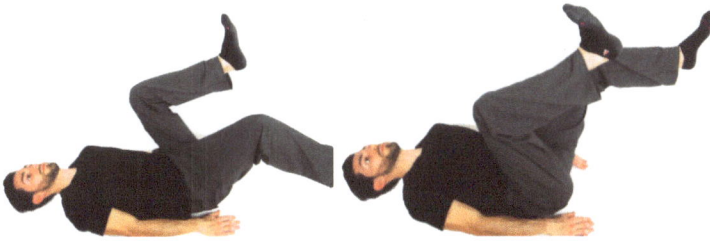

F - 26

Rehabilitation: Early stage
Begin with F-13 & F-14
Rehabilitation: Late stage
Progress to F-5, F-18, F-19 & F-22

LONG TERM

F-6, G-22

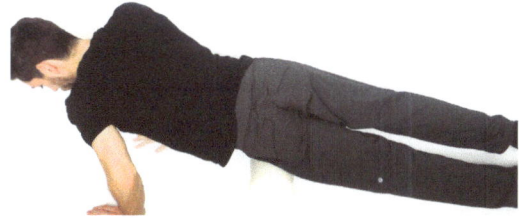

F - 6

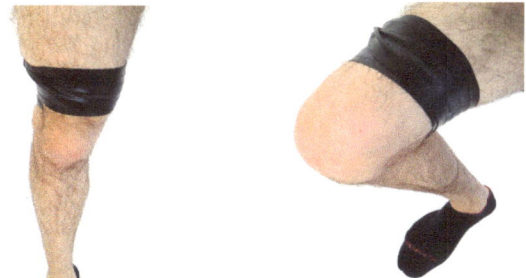

G - 22

123

Legs

Knee arthritis

Arthritis is a well-understood condition, but too often it's poorly managed. I constantly see patients whose experience consists of having pain, visiting their family doctor, having X-rays taken, getting diagnosed as osteoarthritic, picking up a prescription for pain killers and maybe being told to lose some weight.

Arthritis is very manageable and in many cases symptoms can be completely resolved.[25] Unlike in the spine or other parts of the body, the biomechanical operation of the knee is relatively straight forward and can be altered rather specifically. If you've worn down the cartilage in you're knees by putting too much strain on them in unfavorable conditions. Fixing it requires changing the forces going through your knees and making the conditions surrounding them more favorable. People with knee arthritis tend to have weak quadriceps or imbalances in the muscle groups of the thigh.[26]

Stretch certain muscles, strengthen others, wear good footwear, vary the extent and increase the diversity of your activities and supplement with the biochemical building blocks of cartilage. The human body is capable of phenomenal recoveries, as long as YOU give it the opportunity by changing the conditions. That's the difference between someone who will suffer greatly from arthritis and someone who will live without symptoms; the former accepts the diagnosis from their doctor as

an inevitable affliction and does little about it, the latter takes ownership of the issue and puts the effort in to changing the state of their body. It certainly is easier to do this with the support and guidance of knowledgeable therapists, trainers, doctors, physiotherapists and friends. Remember that the amount of improvement you can make is almost fully dependent on the amount of effort you are willing to invest.

It can be important and very helpful to take certain supplements to aid in your recovery. Supplements helpful for knee arthritis are listed at the end of this chapter under Osteoarthritis.

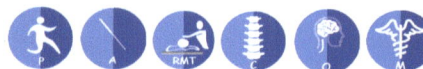

SUGGESTED TREATMENT

SHORT TERM

Muscle tension issues must be addressed first. If you imagine the knee to be a puppet and the muscles all around the thigh to be the puppet strings, you can imagine that pulling one string (muscle) tighter than the rest will have a negative effect on the puppet (knee joint). Firmly push into each muscle along its entire length and determine tight and tender points. Once you've identified which muscles are tight and have trigger points, work them out. Using a foam roller to roll on is more effective than stretching because it is more specific. It is important to ensure the quality of your footwear. Consult the section in this book on Choosing Good Footwear.

Movement imbalances can be hard to pick up, most of the time they are subtle and we are unaware of them. It is valuable to be screened for functional movement imbalances, especially if one knee is worse than the other. A physician or chiropractor specialized in sports is well suited to identify and treat imbalances. It is also important to consider issues in the ankles or hips (usually from old injuries) that can be contributing excess strain on one or both knees.

Use G-22, G-13 and F-26 to reduce tension in the thigh muscles and mobilize the knee joint.

Rehabilitation: Early stage
Begin with F-14, F-4 & H-12
Rehabilitation: Late stage
Progress to F-18, F-19, G-23 & H-14

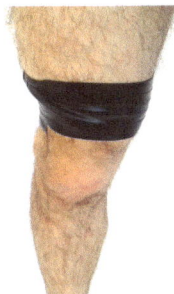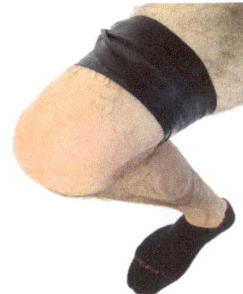

G - 22

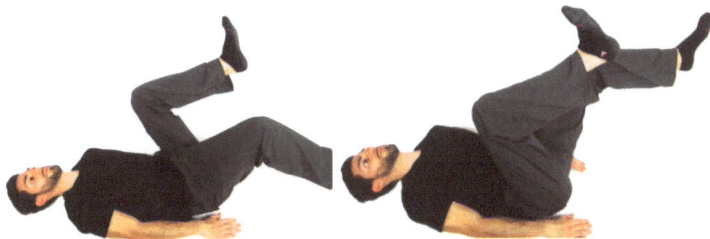

F - 26

LONG TERM

F-6, F-23

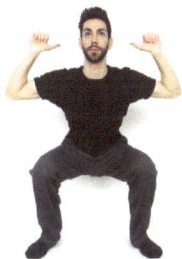

F - 4

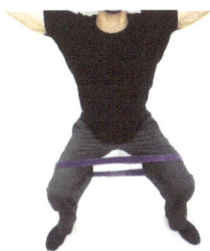

F - 14

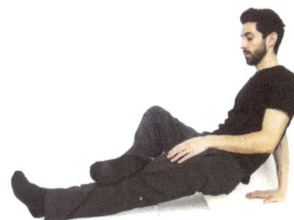

F - 23

Legs

Ankle sprain

Although ankle sprains are not specific to hairstylists, they are so common I thought it would be useful to include some guidance on recovering from one.

If your sprain is serious and any of the following apply to you, then see a doctor immediately: you are over 55 years old, if you heard a loud pop or snap sound, you are unable to walk 4 successive steps, you have severe tenderness directly on the main ankle 'bumps' on either side. This is important to rule out fractures or fully torn ligaments (and based on guidelines called the 'Ottawa Ankle Rules').

If your sprained ankle bruises significantly, swells or is very painful to walk on after a couple days, I also recommend seeing a family doctor or chiropractor. They can order X-rays or ultrasounds to rule out more serious damage. It is very important to be diligent in properly managing it, as an improperly healed ankle can become a chronic issue rather easily.

For the first 36 hours, keep your affected leg elevated and ice 4 times (each time - 10 minutes on, 10 minutes off, 10 minutes on). If you have access to a physiotherapist, chiropractor or sports therapist, a good tape job can help protect the ankle from further injury. A well-fitted ankle brace will also be very useful. Make sure to wear sturdy footwear and definitely avoid heels. Now the rehabilitation - do NOT skip this part. It takes some work but this is the step that prevents the injury from becoming a chronic issue. I have seen too many people who suffer for years from relatively simple ankle sprains because they didn't do any rehab exercises.

Once the pain and swelling have subsided (typically 24-72 hours post injury), begin the following:

Day 1-3:

Use the ankle as much as you want but avoid aggressive activities and ice and elevate after extensive use.

Sitting ankle alphabet exercise - trace out each of the 26 letters of the alphabet with your big toe in the air. Perform twice a day.

Wear a properly fitted ankle brace.

Spend a moderate amount of time walking and swimming in a pool.

Move on the next stage only if you can walk pain-free.

Day 4-10: Do NOT stop rehabilitation efforts when your pain resolves.

Take off ankle brace. Still only wear very supportive footwear.

Proceed to jog, cycle, row, swim or work as much as you would normally.

Put a Theraband around your forefoot, attach the other end to something sturdy and do 20 repetitions of each ankle movement; outwards, inwards, tilting, up and down.

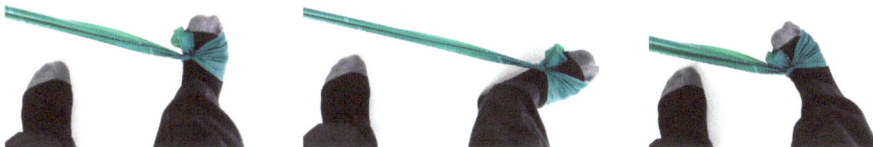

Begin performing 50 daily toe raises daily.

Stand and balance on the affected leg for 60 seconds twice each day. This balance exercise is very important for your recovery.

Day 11-30:

If you have specific activities you would like to attempt (like sports, squats, running, etc.), do so cautiously and less intensely than normal. Wear ankle support. Cease wearing it three weeks after injury, as beyond this it will delay a full recovery. Balance on a wobble board for 5 minutes each day (H-12)

Upgrade to performing the single-leg balance exercise (H-13). If you are keen, buy yourself a 'wobble board' and do sets of 60 second balance exercises every day.

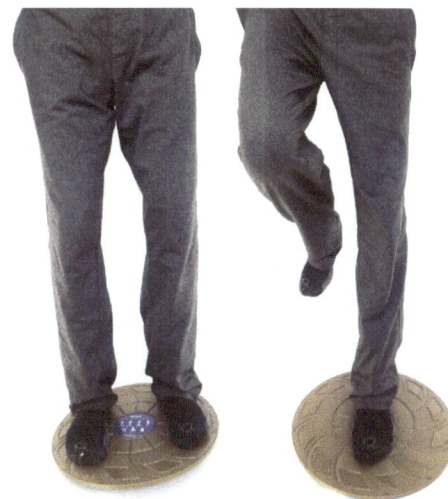

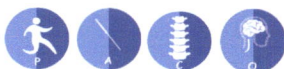

Tip: the research suggests value in supplementing vitamin C (1000-3000 mg/day), vitamin E (400 IU/day) and bromalain (1000-2000 mg/day) while recovering. [27]

Legs

Flat feet

A lot of misconceptions surround the significance of being 'flat footed'. The bottom line is that having flat feet is not a problem in and of itself. This section should be labeled 'sore feet' but people tend to identify themselves as having problematic flat feet. Whether your feet have high arches or appear flat is of only relative importance, the significance should be considered taking into account the rest of your anatomical features as well as your behavior and symptoms. Both high and low arches can be good, depending on what you want to do with those feet. Consider the arches of the feet to be like springs. High arches are like tightly coiled, stiff springs and flat feet are more like loosely coiled dampened springs. Kind of like the difference between driving a racing car (high arches) versus a Cadillac (low arches). With a lot of heavy impact activity, people with high arches generally experience excess strain in knees, hips and the low back and people with flat feet get sore feet more easily. So unless you are a 100-meter sprinter, somewhat flat feet are probably better to have as they spare the rest of your body excess strain. *But* flat-footed folk *are* more likely to strain their feet. Your body is incredibly smart and well designed, so I generally recommend avoiding special footwear sold especially for pronators (another word for flat footed).. at least at first. Solid footwear with generally supportive features (see section on sore feet a few pages back) is sufficient for most and promises

of shoes improving the way your feet work is often more a sales pitch than a statement of clinical value.

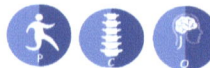

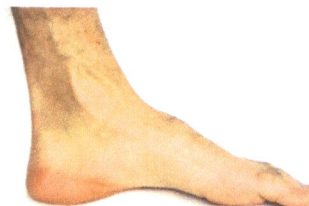

High Arch

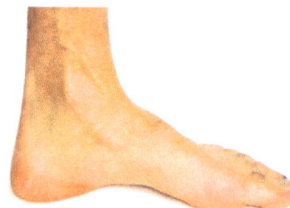

Medium Arch

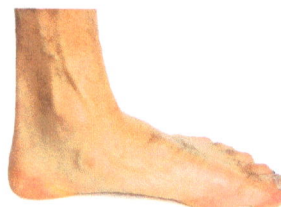

Low Arch

SUGGESTED TREATMENT

SHORT TERM

Make an effort to improve your footwear. Refer to the chapter on Choosing Good Footwear. Take epsom salt baths when your feet are sore, consider using kinesiology tape to help support your feet for a few days at a time. Insoles and custom orthotics are also helpful for those with chronically sore feet. Use G-2 & G-5 to self-treat tired joints and muscles.

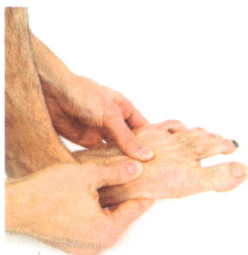 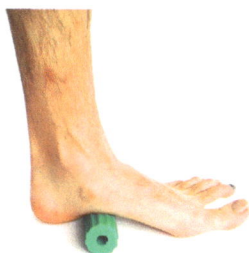

G - 5   G - 2

Rehabilitation: Early stage
Begin with G-6
Rehabilitation: Late stage
Progress to G-21 & H-12

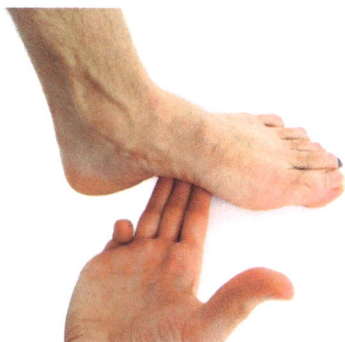 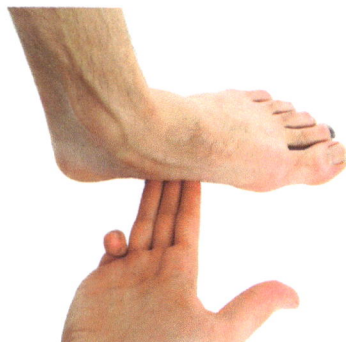

LONG TERM

Reduce the tension in the deepest muscles of the feet using G-17.

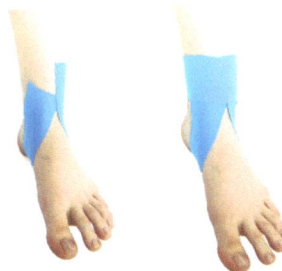

Wrap kinesiology tape around the bottom of the foot at 50% tension, then apply a support piece around the top of the ankle.

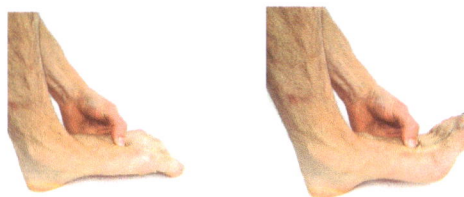

G - 17

Three-finger self-test: Standing upright with your weight on both feet equally, slide three fingers as far into the inside arch of your foot as you can. If you can slide your fingers past the first set of finger creases, it generally means you have medium to high arches. If you don't get up to the first set of finger creases, it means you likely have low arches.

129

General

Osteoarthritis

The joints of our body are robust and can tolerate a good deal of abuse. Generally, arthritic joints are joints that are deteriorating much faster than normal because of a chronic imbalance that causes them to be overloaded consistently in specific ways. A variety of factors can contribute to the imbalance; weight, bone density, nutrition, lifestyle and movement patterns. For those suffering from degenerative arthritis, it is important to work on improving their health comprehensively, though the first step however should be efforts to improve the mechanics of their movement. If someone has arthritic joints, they almost invariably have poor movement patterns and inadequate strength proportions in the muscles of the region.

People suffering from knee arthritis for instance almost always have weakness in specific hip and thigh muscles that support healthy leg movement. Targeting these muscles in strengthening programs will produce consistently significant improvements. Dr. Christopher Powers in California is a world leader in knee rehabilitation, whose work helping people improve their knees is almost always heavily focused on strengthening the hip muscles - the abductors specifically (gluteus medius). I've witnessed great results using his rehabilitation programs in my own practice.

The evidence supporting the use of (specific forms of) nutritional supplementation, low-intensity laser therapy and movement rehabilitation is strong for most types of degenerative arthritis. I therefore advise those concerned about the condition of their joints to consider seeking the support of a range of healthcare providers and therapists.

Nutrition & supplement guidance.[28, 29]

It is important to consult your physician before trying new supplements as there may be contraindications. As an example, glucosamine supplements (one of the most popular and beneficial for sufferers of osteoarthritis) should not be taken by anyone with allergies to shellfish.

Most Effective
Bromelain – In amounts as directed on label or by health care practitioner
Essential fatty acids (omega 3 and omega 6) – As directed on label
Chondroitin sulfate - 500-1000mg daily
Glucosamine sulfate – 500-1000mg daily
Methylsulfoylmethane (MSM) - 500-1000mg 3 times daily

Moderately Effective
S-Adenosylmethionine (SAMe) – 400mg twice daily
Silica – as directed on label
Vitamin E - 200IU daily
Calcium and magnesium - 2000mg and 1000mg respectively, daily
Boron – 3mg with each meal
Niacinamide plus panthothenic acid – 500-1000mg daily

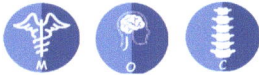

Endnotes

4. Nikita A. Vizniak and Michael A. Carnes, Quick Reference Clinical Chiropractic Conditions Manual, (Location: Professional Health Systems, 2004), page 135.

5. Vizniak and Carnes, Conditions Manual, page 136-137

6. Phyllis A. Balch, Prescription for Nutritional Healing, 4th ed, (New York: Avery, 2006), page 310-311.

7. Francis G. O'Connor, Sports Medicine: Just The Facts. (Location: McGraw-Hill, 2005), page 59-60.

8. Bruce P. Bernard, "Musculoskeletal Disorders and Workplace Factors", National Institute for Occupational Safety and Health (1997)

9. O'Connor, Sports Medicine, page 309.

10. C. Peters-Veluthamaningal, et al. "Corticosteroid Injections Effective for Trigger Finger in Adults in General Practice: A Double-Blinded Randomised Placebo Controlled Trial," Annals of the Rheumatic Diseases 67 (2008): 1262.

11. S. R. Mishra, et al. "Percutaneous A1 Pulley Release by the Tip of a 20-g Hypodermic Needle Before Open Surgical Procedure in Trigger Finger Management," Techniques in Hand Upper Extremity Surgery 17 (2013): 112.

12. J. R. Fowler and M. E. Baratz, "Percutaneous Trigger Finger Release," Journal of Hand Surgery American Volume 38 (2013): 2005.

13. J. Wang, J. G. Zhao, and C. C. Liang, "Percutaneous Release, Open Surgery, or Corticosteroid Injection, Which is the Best Treatment Method for Trigger Digits?," Clinical Orthopaedics and Related Research 471 (2013): 1879.

14. G. I. Bain, and N. A. Wallwork, "Percutaneous A1 Pulley Release a Clinical Study," Hand Surgery 4(1999): 45.

15. G. A. Turowski, P. D. Zdankiewicz, and J. G. Thomson, "The Results of Surgical Treatment of Trigger Finger," Journal of Hand Surgery American Volume 22 (1997): 145.

16. Balch, Prescription for Nutritional Healing, page 585.

17. International Headache Society, "The International Classification of Headache Disorders," Cephalgia 1 (2004)

18. Rami Burstein and Moshe Jakubowski, "Unitary Hypothesis for Multiple Triggers of Pain and Strain of Migraine," Journal of Comparative Neurology 14 (2005): 9-14.

19. Vizniak and Carnes, Conditions Manual.

20. Christina Sun-Edelstein and Alexander Mauskop, "Foods and Supplements in the Management of Migraine Headaches," The Clinical Journal of Pain 25, (2009): 446-52.

21. S. Haldeman and S. Degenais, "Choosing a Treatment for Cervicogenic Headache: When? What? How much?," The Spine Journal 10 (2010)

22. T. R. Bilchik, "A Review of Nonvalidated and Complementary Therapies for Cluster Headache," Current Pain Headache Reports, 8 (2004): 157-61.

23. G. Nicholson and J. Gaston, "Cervical Headache," Journal of Orthopaedic & Sports Physical Therapy 31 (2001): 184-193.

24. Balch, Prescription for Nutritional Healing, pages 217-219

25. C. Ding, et al., "Association of Prevalent and Incident Knee Cartilage Defects with Loss of Tibial and Patellar Cartilage: A Longitudinal Study," Arthritis & Rheumatism 52 (2005): 3918–3927. doi: 10.1002/art.21474

26. J. J. Stefanik et al., "Quadriceps Weakness, Patella Alta, and Structural Features of Patellofemoral Osteoarthritis," Arthritis Care and Research 63 (2011): 1391–1397. doi: 10.1002/acr.20528

27. Vizniak and Carnes, Conditions Manual, page 261.

28. Balch, Prescription for Nutritional Healing, pages 218-221.

29. Vizniak and Carnes, Conditions Manual, pages 366-369.

8

Preventive Exercise

"Smile: Happiness Is Right Under Your Nose!"

- Mary Anne Puleio

PREVENTATIVE EXCERCISE

The single best way to stay physically healthy and injury free throughout your career is to actively inrease your physical capacity in specific ways to buffer the specific demands you have on your body.

The primary purpose of exercise is to develop your strength. An increase in certain forms of strength will allow you to better withstand the strains of your work and maintain a balanced body. The value of stretching is similar but more specific. When you use certain muscles a lot, they get tight, tender and can shorten. Stretching helps lengthen and relax overused muscles. It is most reasonable to do strengthening activities in your own time and stretch at work. The strengthening will build your tolerance to handle your work strains and the stretching will buffer the constant tension your muscles tolerate.

I have carefully considered the elements of functional strength that contribute most significantly to maintaining a healthy body as a hairstylist. The three exercises and three stretches below offer the best bang for your buck and everyone can benefit from them.

The three exercises every hairstylist should master are wall angels (B - 1), side-lying glut lifts (f - 2 or F - 13) and 'stir the pot' (H - 5).

Stretches to do at work

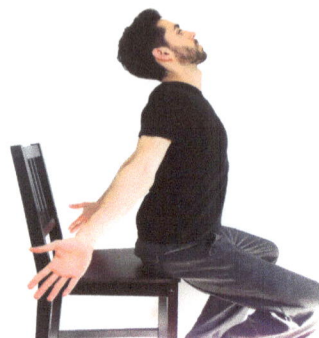

D - 2

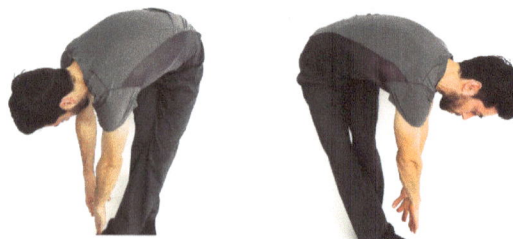

E - 3

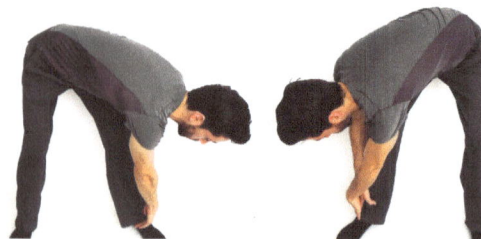

*Refer to Exercise Appendix for descriptions

B - 4

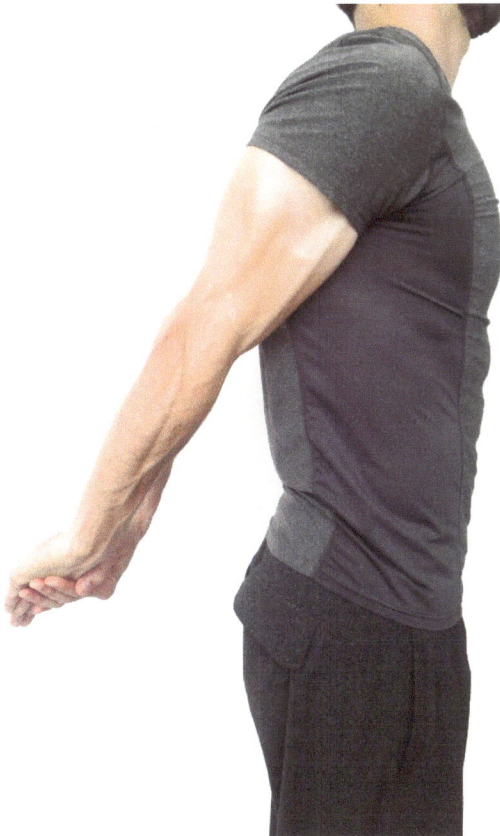

F - 12

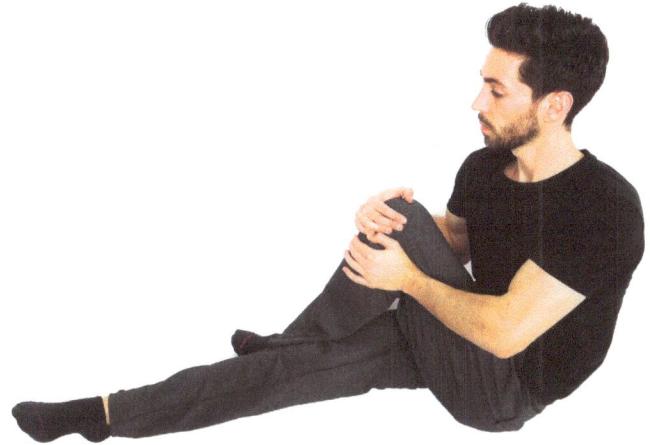

F - 31

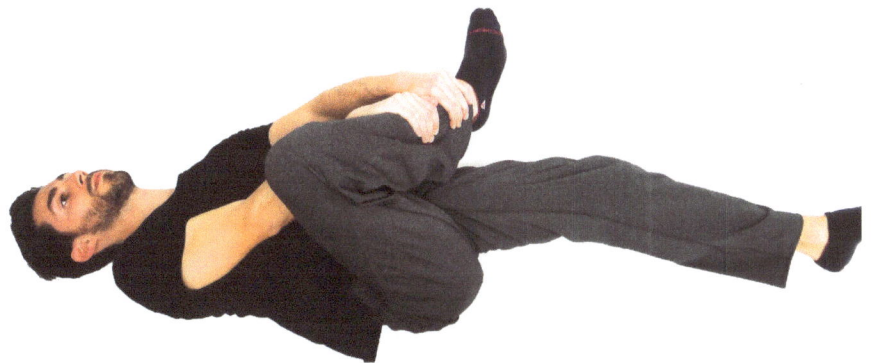

*Refer to Exercise Appendix for descriptions

Preventative exercises to do at home

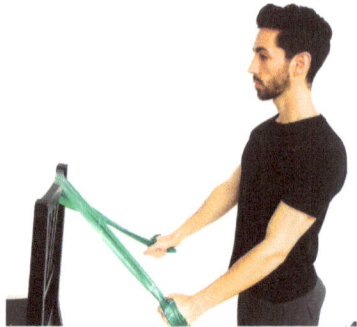

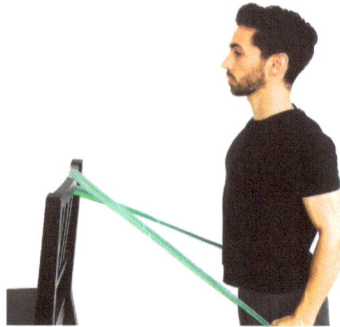

Loop a resistance band around a solid object. Hold either end and pull the band back and down, keeping your elbows straight. Hold your shoulder blades together thoughout the movement. Repeat 30 times.

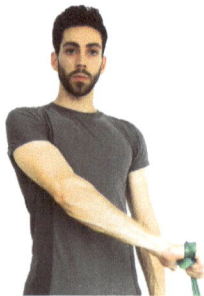

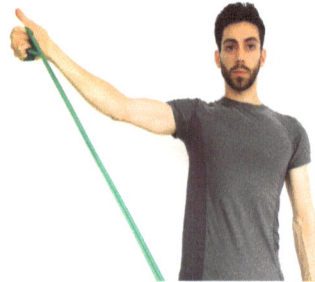

Tie a resistance band to a low object and stand next to it. Using the arm farther away from the object, grab the untied side of the band and slowly pull up and away. Begin the movement with your thumb pointing down and finish with it pointing up. Keep the shoulder blades together the whole time. Repeat 10 times each side.

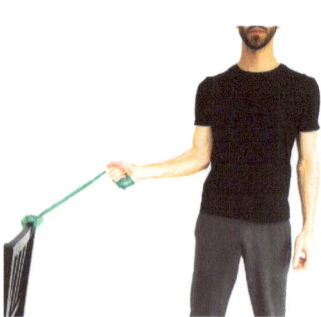

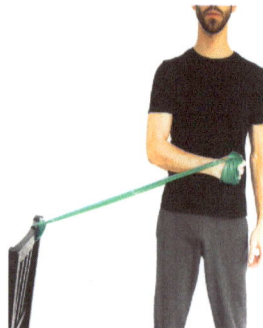

Tie a band to a sturdy object, stand next to it, grab the free end of the band, keep your elbow tucked into your torso and begin with your hand rotated out to be parallel with your elbow. Then slowly rotate your arm across your body without moving your elbow. Slowly return to the original position. Repeat 10 times each side.

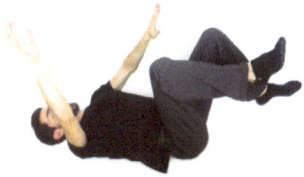

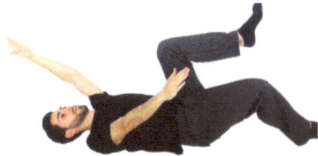

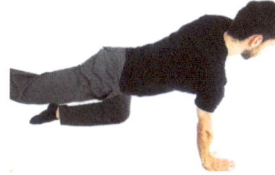

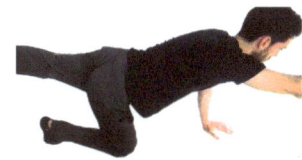

The 'dead bug' and 'bird dog' exercises are among the best ways to improve coordination and strength in your core and low back. To do the 'dead bug': Lie on your back with all limbs up, bring your left arm halfway towards your right leg, then alternate. Ensure slow controlled movement throughout the exercise. Perform for 3 minutes. To do the 'bird dog': starting on all fours, slowly lift one arm and the opposite leg until they are in line with your torso. Keep your core stiff and pelvis straight (don't let it rotate) throughout. 30 lifts each side.

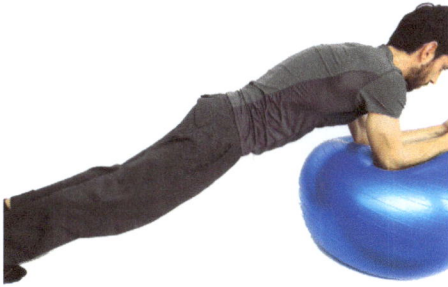

The 'stir the pot' exercise is one of my all-time favourites. As beneficial as it is challenging, it's a powerful way to prevent low back pain. Do a front plank on a yoga ball and make large slow circles with your arms (as though you're stiring a big pot).

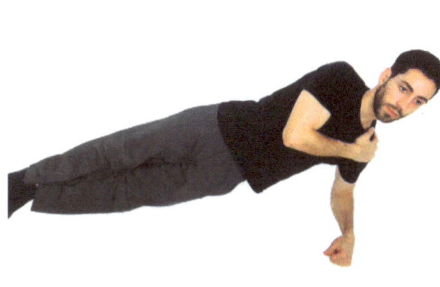

A side plank improves core endurance. Hold yourself up and straight for 10, 20 or 30 second intervals (whichever is reasonable for you). Do 3 repetitions on each side.

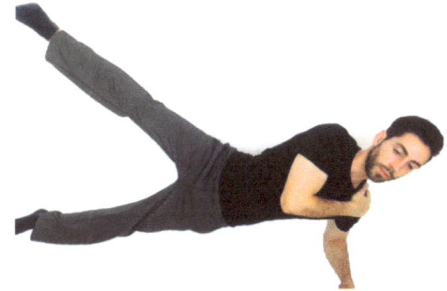

Like 'stir the pot' this is a very advanced exercise. Starting in a side plank position, keep your pelvis forward, lift your leg up high and back a little. Hold it for 10 seconds. Repeat 3 times.

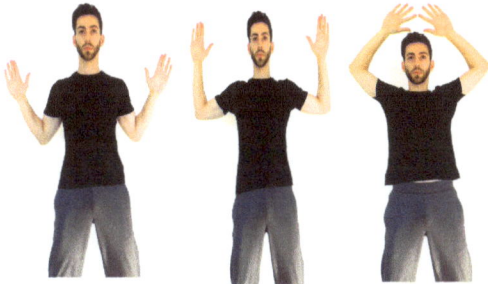

'Wall angels' are great to improve the condition of the shoulders and strengthen the upper back. Lean against a wall and slowly move your hands all the way up and back down without letting your back, wrists or elbows leave the wall. Do sets of 10, twice daily.

The modified crunch is best done with the hands in the small of the low back. Bring your head and shoulders just a bit off the ground and squeeze your abs, holding for 2 seconds. Perform as many as you can.

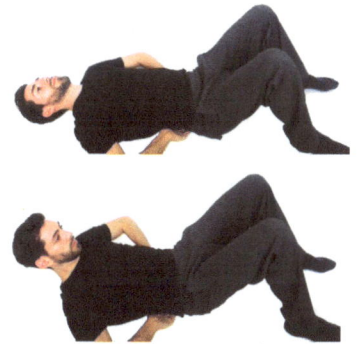

9

Sleep

"Do not go gentle into that good night.
Rage, rage against the dying of the light."
- Dylan Thomas

SLEEP

We all know how important sleep is, but few of us invest in improving the quality of our sleep. Sleeping well is something we are wired to do, but throughout our lives we develop habits and behaviours that impede our body's natural inclinations. For anyone struggling with issues caused by physical strain, it is valuable to exploit the benefits of good restorative sleep to help your body recover properly. Improvements in your sleep quality will also increase your levels of energy, productivity and your overall well being.

Since this book is all about practical solutions, the following set of sleep improvement measures are listed in order of ease of implementation. It's a good idea to start working down the list, taking on the progressively more involved steps until you experience the improvements you are happy with. We won't explore the science of sleep cycles or sleep disorders in this section, but I would encourage anyone keen to improve their health to research the science of sleep to better understand how to affect it. The first steps towards improving sleep should always be to eliminate poor habits. Address the basic behavioural habits that affect your sleep while trying the techniques shared here to improve it. The basics include maintaining somewhat regular sleeping hours, ideally between 6 and 8 hours a night, eating meals at regular and reasonable intervals throughout the day, timing stimulating activities responsibly and avoiding stimulants for several hours before sleep. Those with seriously impeded ability to sleep well despite these things should consider asking their MD for a referral to a sleep clinic and visiting a therapist for Cognitive Behavioural Therapy.

• Calcium and Magnesium supplementation - taking 1500-2000mg of calcium and 1000mg of magnesium daily will help to calm the body and relax the muscles. Take calcium in divided doses, after meals and at bedtime. It is best to use calcium lactate or calcium chelate (avoid lactate if you are sensitive to dairy products). Take the magnesium within a few hours of bed.

• Melatonin supplementation - Melatonin is a hormone your body naturally produces to regulate sleep cycles. Supplementing melatonin can help to modify the onset and quality of sleep. Start with a dose of 1.5mg daily taken 1-2 hours before bed. If not effective, increase the dose gradually up to a maximum of 5mg daily. Do not take it for more than a few weeks at a time, otherwise it will negatively impact your body's ability to regulate it sufficiently.

• Basic breathing meditation - The last 30 minutes before bed should be spent in a relaxed state. Avoid T.V., laptops and phones. Spend 10 minutes with your mind exclusively focused on your breathing. Breath slowly, visualizing your diaphragm moving slowly up and down. Then spend 10 minutes sitting quietly focusing on calming the energies of your body and mind. Move through each part of your body, allowing the muscles to relax. As various thoughts come to mind, let them leave just as quickly and re-focus on relaxing. The last 10 minutes before bed can be spent letting your mind drift, as long as you don't let yourself get worked up.

• Keep your room at about 20 degrees Celsius.

• Eliminate all sources of light in your bedroom - This seems simple, and it is. Many people seem to think there are exceptions to this rule (charging lights on phones, night light, etc.).. there aren't! The receptors in your eyes are stimulated by any form of light, which will interfere with your sleeping.

• Herbal supplements that can help induce and improve sleep include; california poppy, hops, kava kava, chamomile, lemon balm, passionflower, skullcap and valerian root. These herbs, taken before bedtime in either capsule or extract form can improve REM sleep, relax the nervous system and provide a mild sedative effect to help induce sleep. It is wise to rotate among different herbs and avoid extensive use of any one supplement.

• Add complex stabilization activities to your workout - Adding single-leg and single-arm exercises to your routine will tax your nervous system more heavily than typical exercises. As will exercises done on unstable surfaces. Using a wobble-board can be useful. The more challenging to your balance, the better it will work. Kettlebell training can also be great for this.

• Eat a meal heavy in protein and (healthy) fat within 3 hours of bed. It doesn't work for everyone, nor is it healthy for everyone, but it helps some people and may be worth a shot. Foods with tryptophan can help to promote sleep. You can increase your evening intake of bananas, figs, dates, milk, nut butter, tuna, turkey and yogurt.

• Avoid alcohol, nicotine and caffeine in the four to six hours before bedtime. Even though you may feel that they help relax you or induce sleep, they all reduce the quality of sleep.

10

Skin Health

"Your silence will not protect you."

- Audre Lorde

SKIN HEALTH

The majority of hairstylists suffer work-related skin problems at some point, and roughly 20% of hairstylists leave the profession because of skin problems and allergies. This is a preventable problem, but one that you need to be proactive about. Make informed decisions when choosing and using products to minimize the hazards of working with chemicals. Young hairstylists often develop allergic contact dermatitis and experienced hairstylists often develop allergies to formaldehyde. Allergies develop faster in younger workers, which is why it's very important to educate and inform young hairstylists and apprentices about the risks of certain chemicals and how to reduce exposure.

Epidemiological studies done by the National Institute of Occupational Health (NIOSH) have demonstrated an increased risk of cancer among salon workers. Increased risk of bladder cancer and multiple myeloma is tied mostly to the use of dyes, which can be absorbed through the skin. An increased risk of cancer of the larynx in men has been observed and stomach, lung, uterus and ovarian cancer in women in the profession.[25] It is important to consider that these risks can be mitigated by taking measures to protect yourself from exposure to known carcinogens.

Eczema is an inflammatory condition of the skin that has different forms. The term "dermatitis" is often used as a synonym for "eczema". Hand eczema is a common skin disease affecting about 10% of the general working population, but at least 20% of hairstylists. In this context, eczema can also be called occupational contact dermatitis. It is characterized by dryness, itchiness, scaling, flaking, blistering, redness and pain on the skin of the hands. Shampoo is the most commonly used skin irritant. For some, shampooing several clients a day wouldn't irritate the skin of their hands and for others it can cause serious reactions.

Wearing good quality protective gloves when using colour, bleach or wave solutions is a must. A Swedish study found that cutting newly dyed hair contaminates the hands of hairstylists to an extent that justifies either wearing gloves or always cutting hair before dyeing it. [26] Wearing gloves each time you shampoo a client may seem tedious, but well worth it. Gloves should also always be worn when using, handling or transferring chemical products (bleaches, dyes, wave or straightening serums, etc.) and when washing or disinfecting equipment. Drying hands thoroughly after each shampoo and wash helps to prevent excess chemical irritation. Moisturizing after each wash can help prevent the skin from drying out. Using a protectant can be very useful to protect from the irritation of repeated shampooing and other chemical exposures. There are a number of 'invisible glove' products on the market that seem to be a good alternative to wearing gloves but tend to either not work as well as gloves or have significant side-effects. Avoid wearing rings or other jewelry on your hands, as they trap chemicals underneath them and worsen exposure. Skin protection creams are helpful in offsetting the irritation caused by gels, pastes, sprays and other frequently used substances. The more effective creams are those with (5%) aluminum chlorohydrate or beeswax as ingredients. It's always a good idea to use creams free of fragrances and preservatives. The hair industry in the Netherlands and in Germany have stringent workplace guidelines regarding skin protection for hairstylists which entail regular application of water-resistant skin creams and monthly skin checks at salons. They recognized the extent of the problem and made these measures mandatory. If your salon doesn't take such measures, I recommend you implement them yourself and be strict about it.

The most common gloves used by hairstylists include natural latex rubber, nitrile rubber, polyethene and polyvinyl chloride. The quality of a glove isn't only about the material it's made of, but also the manufacturing process. Natural latex gloves are the most commonly used, because they are highly elastic and cheap. Latex is a poor choice in many cases however as latex allergies are not uncommon (which can cause potential reactions for both the stylist and client). Nitrile rubber gloves are a good alternative for this reason as well as the fact that they are quite strong and have good resistance to oils and solvents. Polyethene gloves are thin, not very flexible and are typically porous. Polyvinyl chloride gloves are quite effective at repelling water-based chemicals but are not so resistant to organic solvents.

The way you use gloves is as important as the quality of the gloves in preventing skin contamination. Do not re-use disposable gloves. Put on gloves before beginning the work with chemicals and before handling equipment and workspaces that have been used.

Dealing with dermatitis, eczema or any work-related skin problems requires a reduction in exposure to chemicals, reduction in wet work, better hand protection and the regular use of good natural moisturizing cream.

Endnotes

25. Nellie J. Brown, Health Hazard Manual for Cosmetologists, Hairdressers, Beauticians and Barbers, (New York: Cornell University, 1987

26. Marie-Louise Lind. "Hairdressers –Hand Eczema, Hair Dyes and Hand Protection," THE DEPARTMENT OF WORK AND HEALTH, National Institute for Working Life, Stockholm, Sweden, 2006.

11

Respiratory Health

"Until I feared I would lose it, I never loved to read. One does not love breathing."

- Harper Lee

RESPIRATORY HEALTH

Hairstylists are at higher risk of developing respiratory issues than the average person. Working in a salon means being exposed to higher volumes of dangerous airborne substances that have many possible consequences. The effects of long-term exposure to chemicals in hair products range from a runny nose to cancer. Furthermore, there is now strong evidence linking exposure to chemicals in hair salons to premature births and miscarriages. [27, 28, 29] It is incumbent on YOU to take responsibility for your health in this regard. It is valuable to assume that neither your salon owner nor the product manufacturers are doing all they can to protect your health in this regard. Salon owners should take measures to improve ventilation or screen products for safety, but just assuming they do this adequately may be dangerous. Likewise, product manufacturers should be limiting use of hazardous chemicals to protect hairstylists, but unfortunately they don't always keep strict standards. In my experience very few salons take adequate measures to protect their staff from the dangers of long-term chemical exposure. I encourage you to consult the information in this book, do further research, get in touch with your local health authorities, unions, health & safety committees, start discussions and ask hard questions. Do not make assumptions, don't take someone's word for it and don't be complacent. If you have concerns, express them. Your health is your most valuable asset and improperly managed chemical exposure is a serious threat.

Frequent exposure to chemicals increases the prevalence and risk of developing asthma, chronic bronchitis, allergies and other respiratory illnesses. [30, 31] The following is a list of types of products and the chemicals they contain that are well-known asthmagenic agents (causing asthma and lung irritation):

In shampoos & conditioners - Sericin

In bleach containing products- Persulfates (ex. ammonium, potassium, sodium persulfate)

In hair color & dyes - Monoethanolamine, ethylenediamine, O-toulidine/2-methylaniline (classified carcinogen, 2,4-toluenediamin, resorcinol, m-phenylenediamine, p- aminophenol, m-aminophenol, p-phenylenediamine (this one will almost always be in colour formulas, look for products with lower quantities).

In perming & wave solutions - Ammonia

In hair spray - Polyvinylpyrrolidone (PVP) and sericin

In smoothing serums - Formaldehyde, methylene glycol

Persulfates in bleaches, PVP in hairsprays and formaldehyde in smoothing serums are the most likely culprits of chronic illness among hairstylists. Keratin products are particularly infamous for containing (sometimes illegally) high volumes of formaldehyde and formaldyhyde-producing compounds. The International Agency for Research on Cancer (and many other organizations) have declared formaldehyde a human carcinogen. Formaldehyde-free and ammonia-free keratin products are available on the market. Most governments that have regulations on the matter suggest using keratin products with a maximum formaldehyde content of 0.1 or 0.2%. Yet we still see popular smoothing products with much higher levels.

Many products that don't say 'Formaldehyde' on the labels are still dangerous. The chart "Chemicals That Can Release Formaldehyde" in the appendix is based on information from the US Occupational Health & Safety Administration [32] and lists all chemicals which can release formaldehyde.

Take it upon yourself to know about the products you work with. Look at the labels and MSDS information on dyes, bleaches, smoothing products, and anything you use regularly. Then follow up; look into what these chemical names actually mean and how they might affect you when you use them. Do what you can to avoid extensive use of products that contain the dangerous ingredients. When you do use them, make sure your work area is well ventilated. In the very least, you can always plug in an extra fan nearby if you have doubts. I recommend that you protect yourself by researching the standards of your local health and safety regulatory body and ensuring your workplace meets the standards regarding ventilation. It is also wise to ensure that the products you use frequently are approved for use by your provincial or federal health and safety organization.

Below is a guideline for salon owners based on standards laid out by the (American) Occupational Health and Safety Administration. If products containing formaldehyde are being used, it is their responsibility to ensure the following criteria:

Install and maintain ventilation systems in areas where products are mixed and keep the air levels of formaldehyde below OSHA standards.

Test the air in your salon during product use to determine formaldehyde exposure levels. According to OSHA, the limits are 0.75 parts formaldehyde per million parts of air (ppm) for an 8-hour work shift or the Short Term Exposure Limit (STEL) of 2 ppm during a 15-minute period. You must then notify salon workers of air testing results.

Provide respirators and written posted warnings if air levels of formaldehyde exceed the limits.

Test air quality at least every 6 months when levels are at or above 0.5 ppm and every 12 months if levels are at or above 2 ppm.

Use work practices that may reduce exposures, such as reducing the heat settings on blow dryers and flat irons.

Provide workers with all necessary protective equipment including gloves, face shields, chemical splash goggles and chemical-resistant aprons. Train workers how to use equipment when mixing and applying products.

Explain to workers how to read and understand information on product labels and MSDS. Ensure the workplace has eye and skin washing equipment.

Inform workers about the health effects of formaldehyde (including signs and symptoms of exposure), how to use products safely, on the use of protective equipment, cleaning up spills and proper disposal of products and contaminated clothing. Training should be done upon hiring and annually thereafter.

Prepare a written hazard communication program that describes how workers will be informed about labels, warnings, MSDSs and training requirements.

Offer workers the appropriate medical attention if they develop signs and symptoms of formaldehyde exposure.

Keep records of air quality testing,

Endnotes

27. W. M. Kersemaekers, N. Roeleveld, and G. A. Zielhuis, "Reproductive Disorders Due to Chemical Exposure Among Hairdressers," Scandinavian Journal of Work, Environment and Health 21 (1995)

28. C. Peters, M. Harling, and M. Dulon, "Fertility Disorders and Pregnancy Complications in Hairdressers – A Systematic Review," Journal of Occupational Medicine and Toxicology 5 (2010): 24.

29. V. Baste et al., "Infertility and Spontaneous Abortion Among Female Hairdressers: The Hordaland Health Study," Occupational and Environmental Medicine 50 (2008)

30. E. Mounier-Geyssant, et al., "Exposure of Hairdressing Apprentices to Airborne Hazardous Substances," Environmental Health: A Global Access Science Source 5 (2006)

31. M. Akpinar-Elci, A. Cimrin, and O. Elci, "Prevalence and Risk Factors of Occupational Asthma Among Hairdressers in Turkey," Journal of Occupational and Environmental Medicine 44 (2002): 585.

32. Occupational Safety and Health Administration, "Hair Salons: Facts About Formaldehyde in Hair Products; Formaldehyde in Your Products," Accessed March 16, 2014, https://www.osha.gov/SLTC/hairsalons/formaldehyde_in_products.html

12

Helpful Tools

This list is just a sampling of some tools that can be helpful.

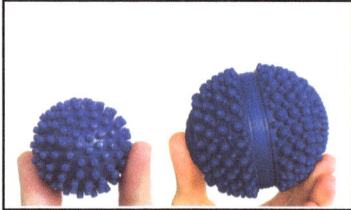

Acuball mini & Acuball

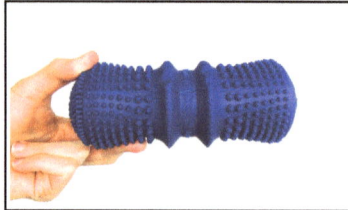

Acuback

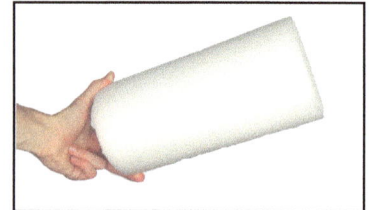

Foam roller

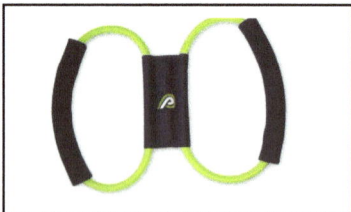

Posture support bands

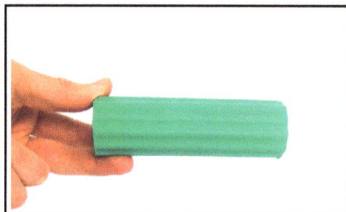

Theraband foot roller

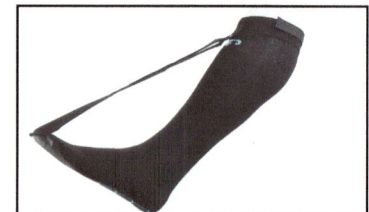

Tension sock for plantar fasciitis

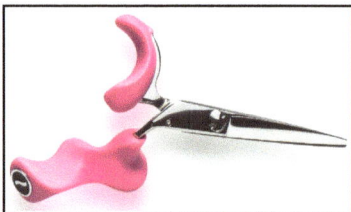

Exthand shears

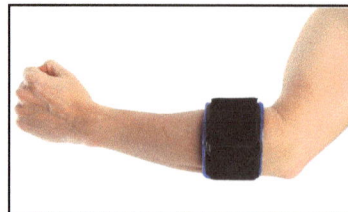

Tennis/golfers elbow strap

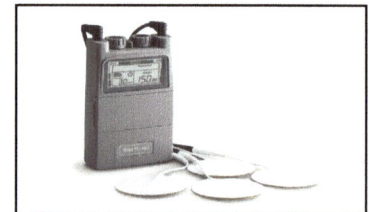

TENs unit

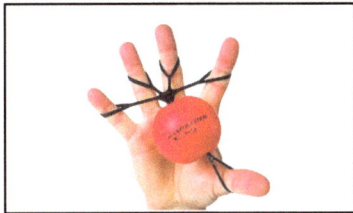
Handmaster plus

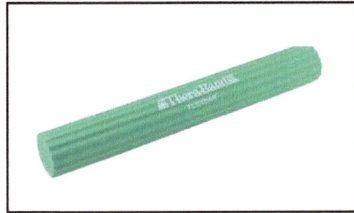
Theraband bar

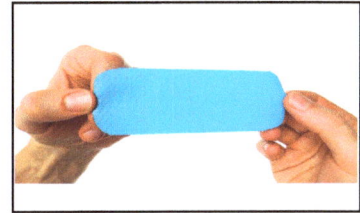
Kinesiology tape

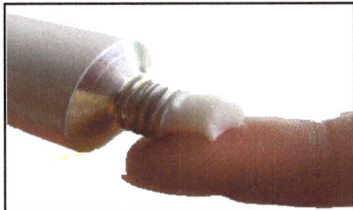
Muscle pain cream

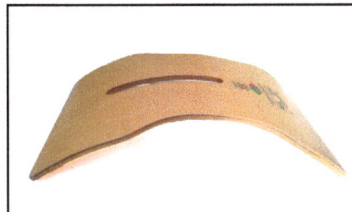
Back bridge

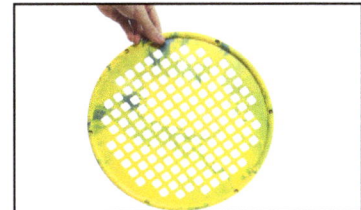
Power Web

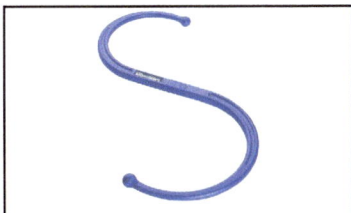
Backnobber

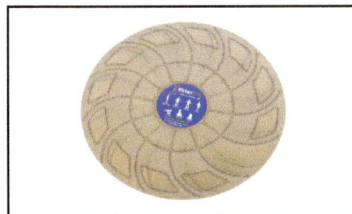
Wobble Board

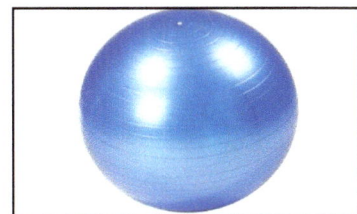
Yoga/Swiss Ball

5 - Minute Plan For The Sore Neck

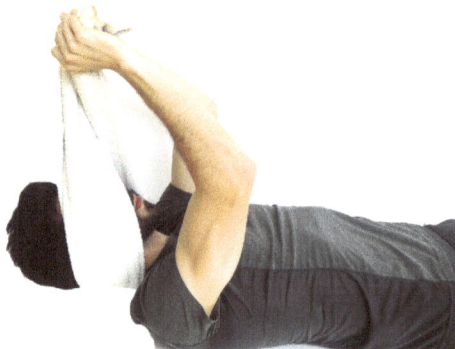

Wrap a folded up towel around the top of your neck and hold either side. Lie down, make sure it supports the base of your skull so that your head doesn't tilt backwards. Cross the towel in your grip, then gently oscillate your head from side to side, focusing on letting your neck muscles turn off.

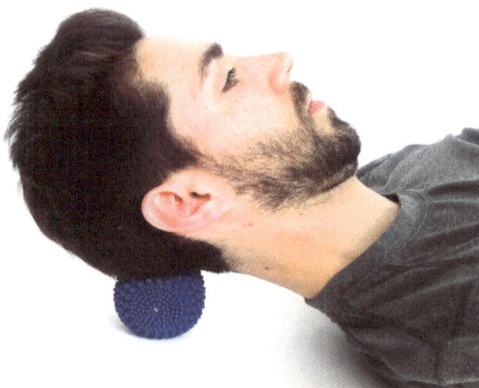

Using a heated regular sized acuball, line the middle ridge up with the middle of your neck (the spine). Tuck your chin and line the ball up so that it rests at the base of your skull, right where it starts to become tender. Take several slow deep breaths, allowing the weight of your head to sink into the ball with each breath out.

Stretch your trapezius muscles thoroughly by sitting on one hand with your palm up. Get your hand underneath you enough that you can't raise that shoulder. Then use the other arm to pull your head gently to the opposite side. Hold for 30 seconds each side.

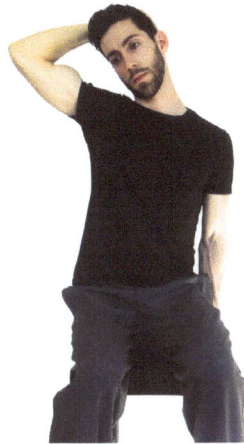

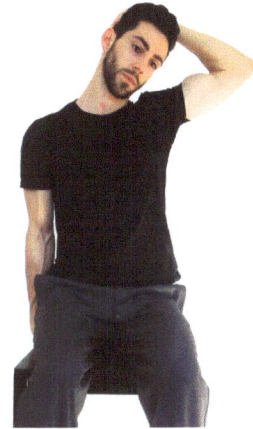

Similar to the trapezius stretch, sit on your hand with the palm up, ensuring that you can't raise the shoulder. Then use the other hand to gently pull the head down while rotating your head to the opposite direction. Hold for 30 seconds on each side.

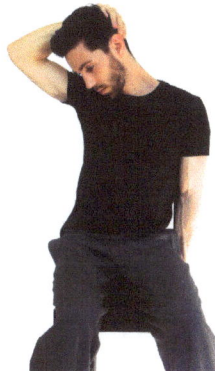

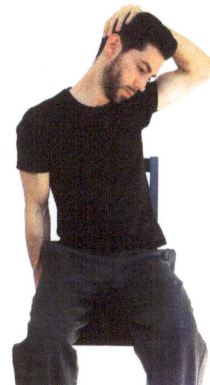

5 - Minute Plan For The Sore Upper Back

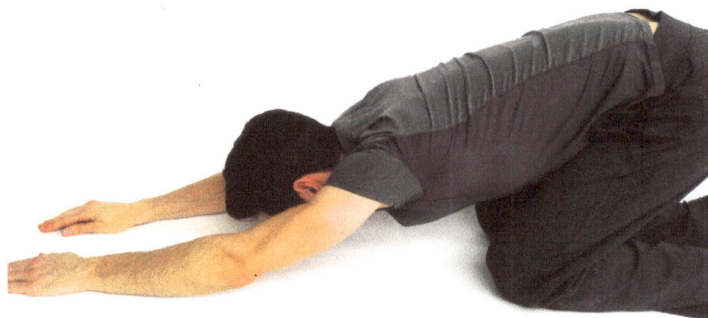

Childs pose is a great way to undo tension built up in the middle back. Start on your knees, lean forward with arms outstretched, reach forward and lower your head as you breathe slowly and deeply. Allow your shoulders to get lower and farther from your torso with each breath.

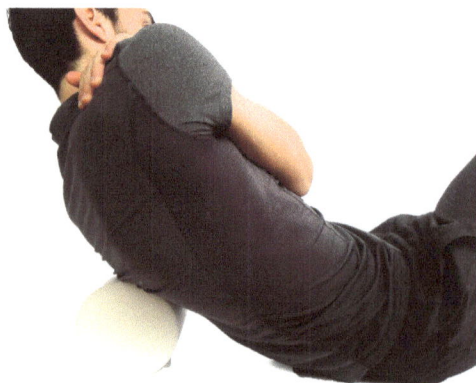

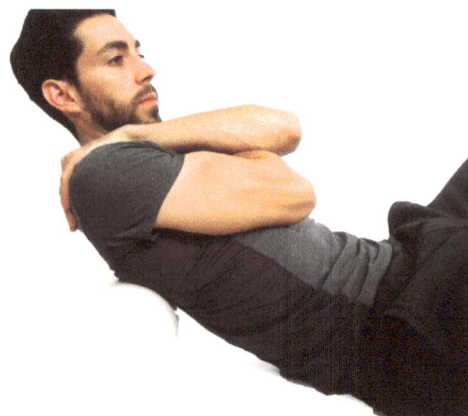

Using a foam roller for the back should be done cautiously. Preferably on a mat or carpet, gently roll from your mid to upper back on each side, avoiding rolling on the spine.

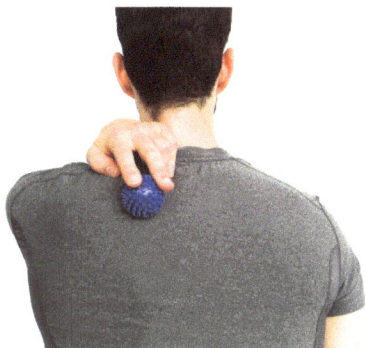

Place an acuball mini between the spine and shoulder blades, push up against a wall, lean into the ball and slowly roll up and down on each side.

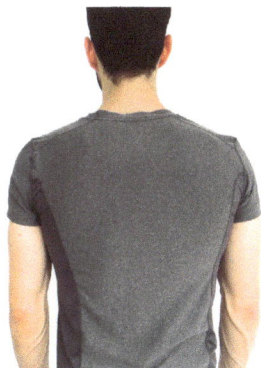

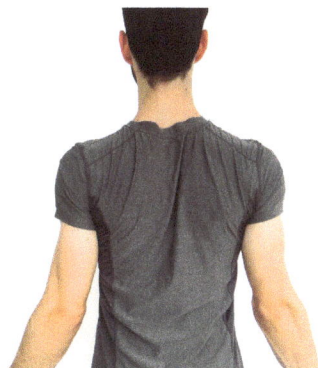

Rotate your hands out so that your palms face forward, roll your shoulders all the way back and then all the way down. Hold for 3 seconds. Repeat 10 times.

5 - Minute Plan For The Sore Lower Back

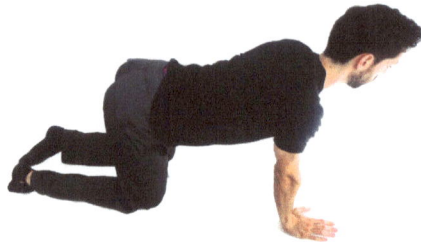

On your hands and knees, take a deep breath in and let your belly relax and sink towards the floor as you exhale. Hold for 3 seconds.

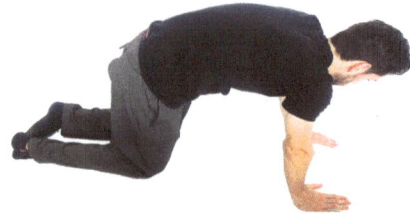

As you breath deeply in, raise the middle of your spine towards the ceiling as high as you can and hold for 3 seconds. Move very slowly. Repeat for at least 1 minute.

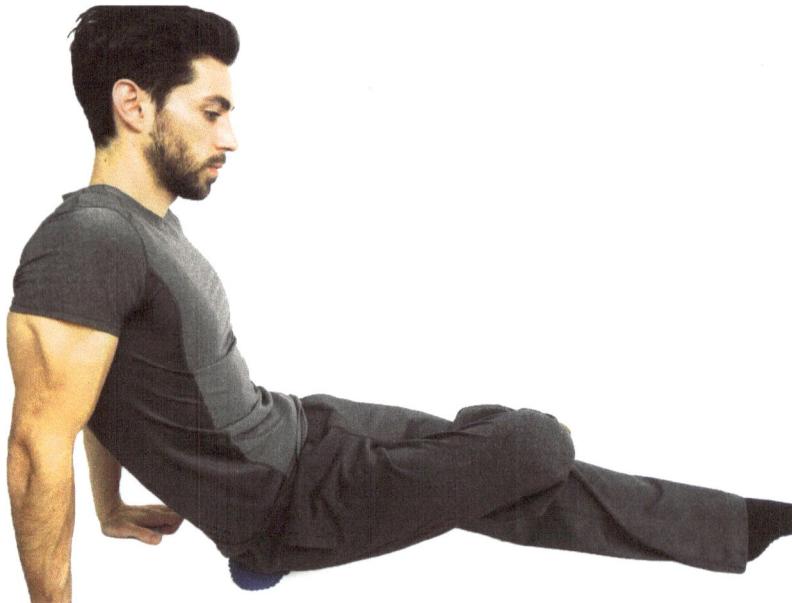

Roll slowly and carefully over a ball or foam roller (I prefer using a heated acuball). Keep your leg bent and crossed over the other leg and use your arms to roll your glutes slowly over the ball. When you find a particularly tight and tender spot, hold it for 15 seconds. Roll for 30 seconds on each side.

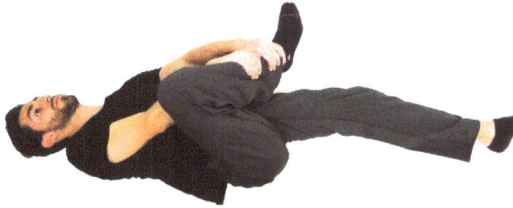

Lying on your back, hold your leg with both hands just above the ankle and bring your foot towards your head. You should feel the stretch in your gluteal muscles. Hold the stretch for 30 seconds on each side.

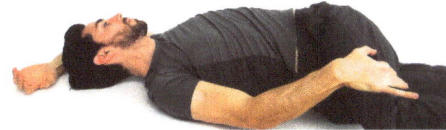

OR

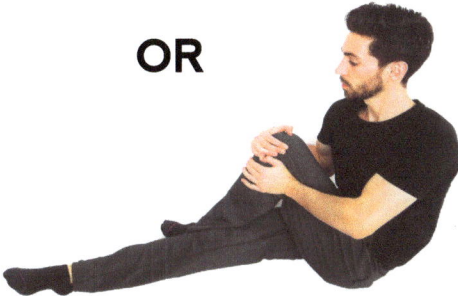

Alternatively, cross one leg over the other while sitting and pull your whole leg towards your chest, keeping the foot above the other knee. Hold the stretch for 30 seconds on each side.

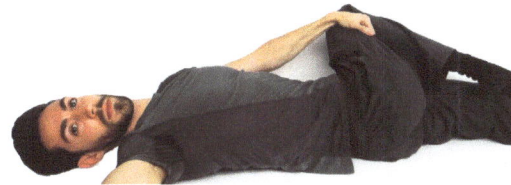

OR

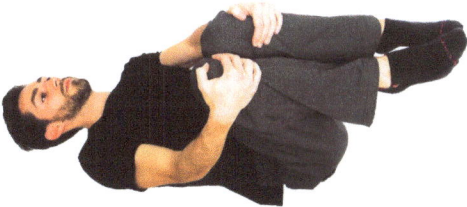

Lying on your back, bring both knees towards your chest and hold the stretch for 30 seconds.

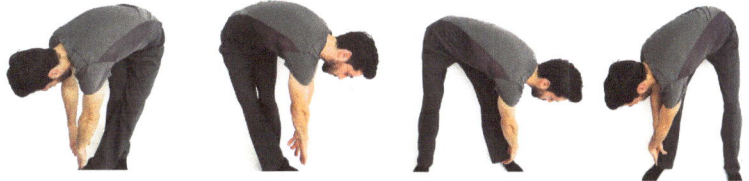

Twisting at the middle of your torso, keep one shoulder on the ground and reach the leg of the same side to the opposite side and touch the knee to the floor. Hold for 30 seconds.

While twisting, use your free arm to gently bring the knee closer to the ground.

Stretch your QL muscles either by just reaching down to your toes to each side or crossing one leg over the other and then reaching for the bottom of your foot.

Exercise Appendix

A - 1

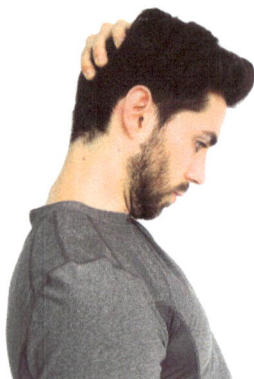

Tuck your chin while gently pulling your head down with your hand. Hold for 20 seconds.

A - 2

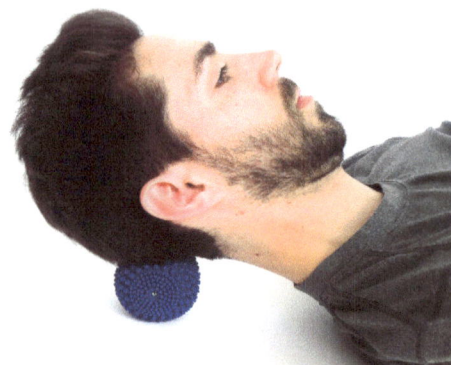

Line up the groove in the Acuball with the middle of your spine. Tuck your chin and nudge the ball right up to the tender points at the base of your skull. Keep your chin tucked and allow your head to relax. Wait until the pressure subsides, usually between 30 seconds to 3 minutes.

A - 3

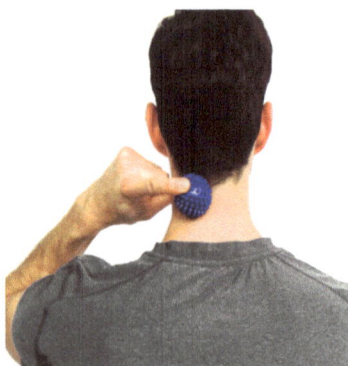

Line the ball up to one side at the base of your neck. Lie on it until the pressure is sufficient.

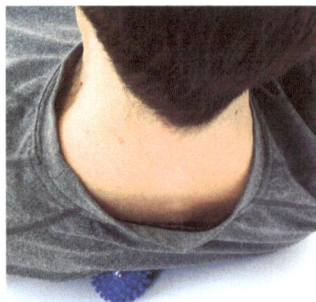

Slowly raise and lower your head 10 times.

A - 4

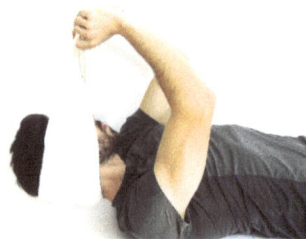

Hold both ends of a towel folded lengthwise. Set the middle of the towel under the base of your head carefully. It should feel like you can support the full weight of your head with your towel.

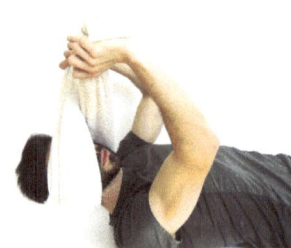

Practice small movements until you are able to relax all your neck muscles, supporting your head only with your hands. Then use the towel to slowly rotate your head to each side. 1-5 minutes.

A-5

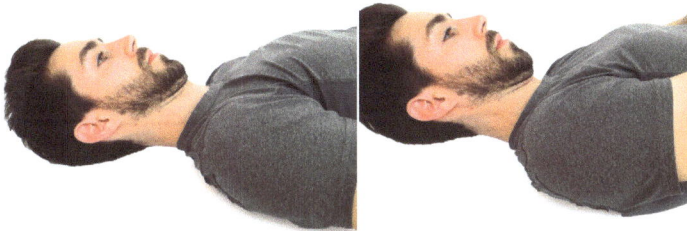

Lying flat on your back, tuck your chin fully. Hold your head an inch off the ground, keeping your chin tucked.

Hold it for as long as you can until you begin to shake. Keep track of the time and use it as your baseline. Repeat the hold 3 times. Work towards 30 seconds.

A-6

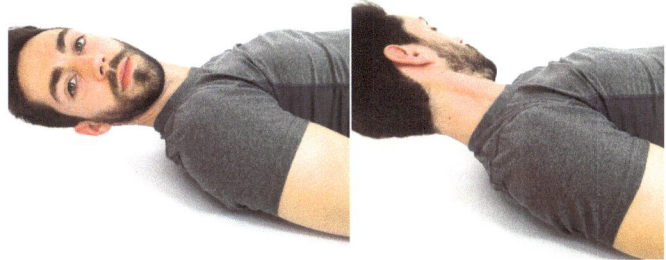

Lying on your back, tuck your chin and lift your head slightly off the ground.

Slowly rotate your head to both sides, keeping your chin fully tucked. Rotate to each side 6 times, then repeat.

A-7

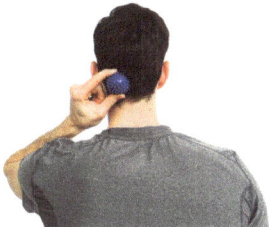

Find the tender area just below the ridge of the skull. Use either a small ball on both sides or a large acuball centered along the spine.

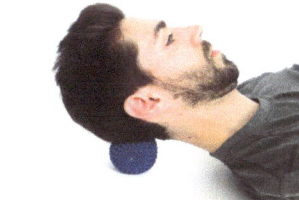

Keep the chin tucked, relax the weight of your head to increase the pressure. Allow the tension to dissipate over a few minutes.

A-8

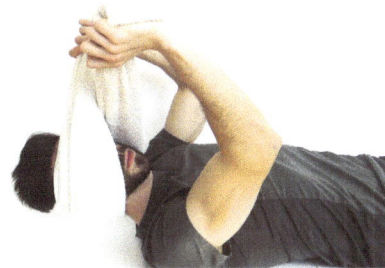

Wrap a folded towel around the back of your head and hold both ends. Tuck your chin and gently pull your neck up to stretch the muscles at the base of your skull. Hold the stretch for 30 seconds.

A - 9

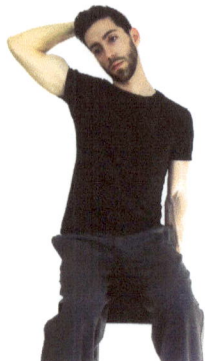

Sitting on the palm of your hand so that you can't lift your shoulder, use the other hand to pull your head gently to the other side.

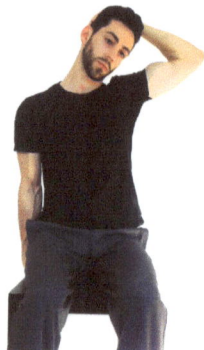

Stretch the trapezius on both sides. 3 times for 30 seconds each.

A - 10

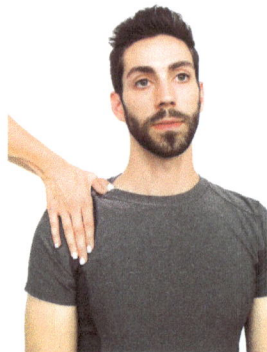

Have a friend hold a thumb firmly into the spot in between the shoulder blade and collar bone.

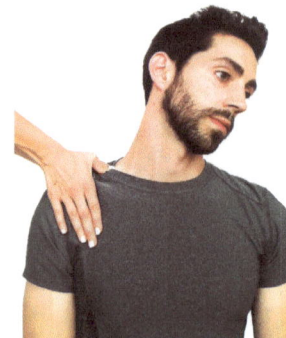

While the pressure is maintained, stretch your head to the opposite side and hold for 15 seconds. Repeat 4 times each side.

A - 11

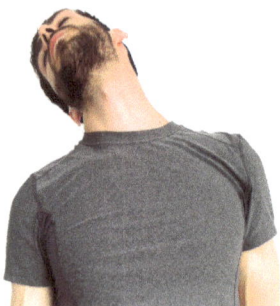

Stretch your SCM muscle by tilting your head back, tilted to one side and rotated to the same side.

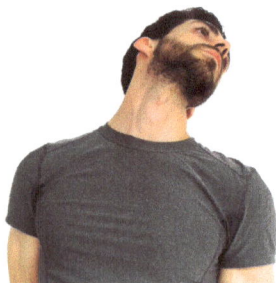

Stretch both sides for 20 seconds each. Repeat twice for each side.

A - 12

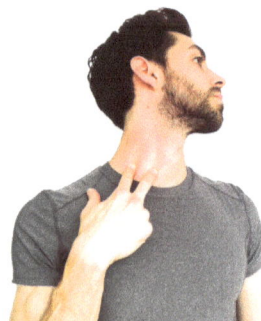

To intensify the SCM stretch, push a finger one either side of the muscle and pull down firmly while you perform the A - 11 stretch.

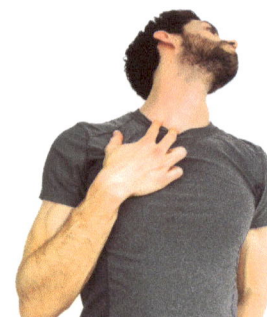

Be careful not to push on the carotid artery. Stretch for 10 seconds and repeat 4 times on each side.

A - 13

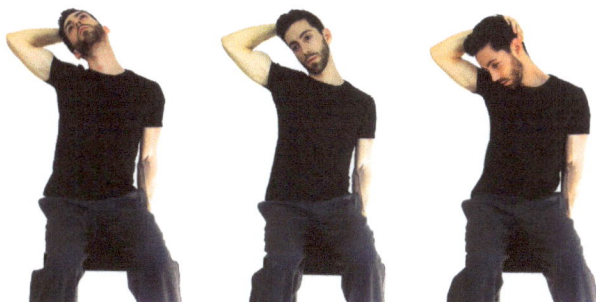

Stretch the anterior scalene by sitting on your palm, rotating the head back towards the lowered arm & tilting the head away.

The middle scalene is stretched by just tilting your head away while sitting on the opposite palm.

The posterior scalene is stretched by tilting the head away & rotating to the opposite side while pulling the head down and sitting on the opposite palm.

A - 14

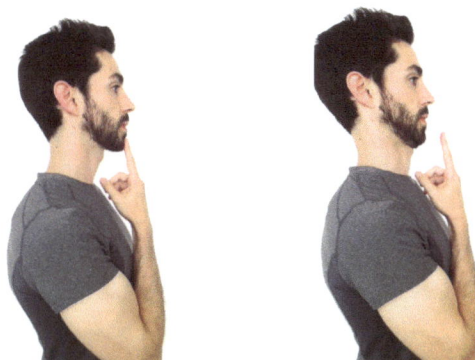

Place your finger on your chin.

Without moving your finger, tuck your chin as far back away from the finger as possible without moving the rest of your body. Hold for 10 seconds. Repeat 8 times.

B - 1

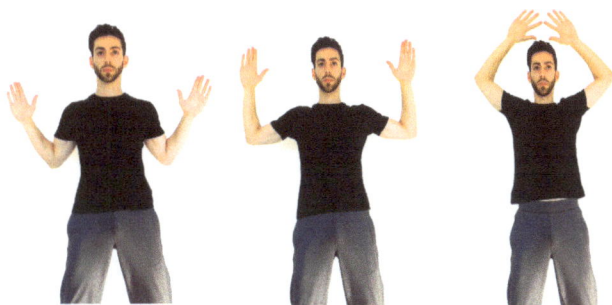

Stand with your back, elbows and wrists against a wall. Slowly raise your arms all the way up until the fingers touch WITHOUT letting the elbows or wrists leave the wall. Repeat 10 times.

B - 2

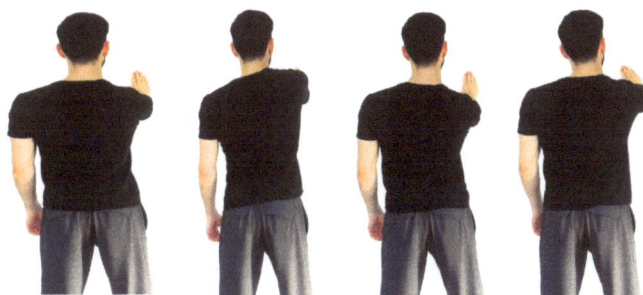

Place your palm on a wall and keep your elbow straight. Move your shoulder up, down, to the right and left slowly. Explore the full range of motion without bending the elbow, moving your torso or hand off the wall. Repeat one full set 6 times.

173

B - 3

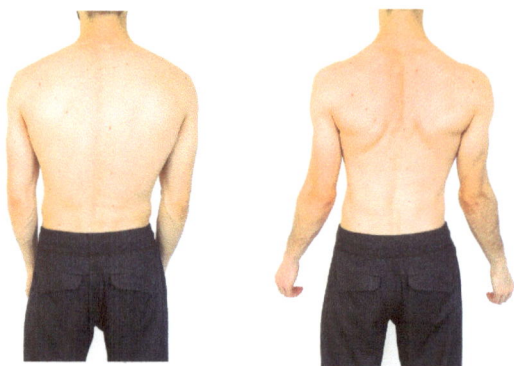

Pull your shoulder blades back and down.
Hold for 10 seconds. Repeat 10 times.

B - 4

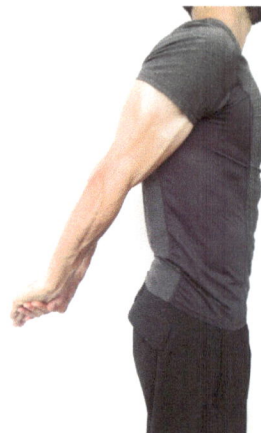

Clasp your hands together behind your
back and slowly reach as far back as you
can while pushing your chest forward.

B - 5

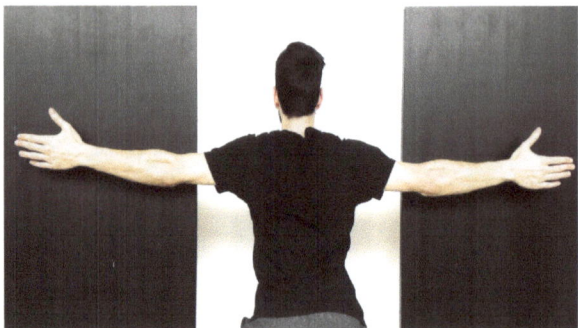

Spread arms strait out, move partially through a
doorway, letting your arms be held back while your
torso moves forward, stretching your pectorals.

B - 6

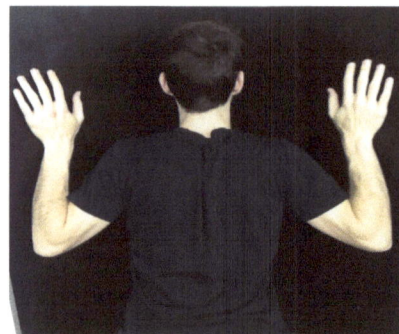

An alternative pectoral stretch is to use the
corner of a room. Lift arms up to 90 degrees,
bend the elbows and walk right up to the
corner, moving your torso forwards.

B-7

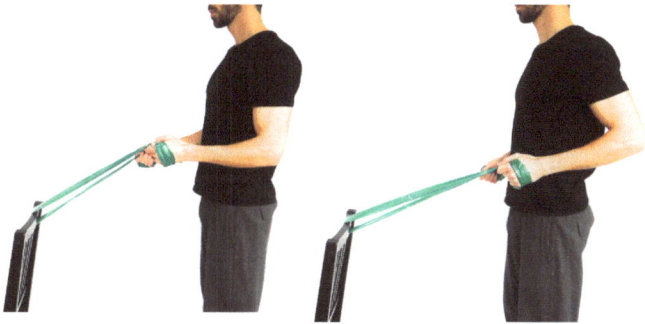

With a resistance band looped through a sturdy object, reach slightly forward and take a step back. Slowly pull your arms and shoulders backwards.

Release the tension slowly to the original position. Perform 3 sets of 15 reps.

B-8

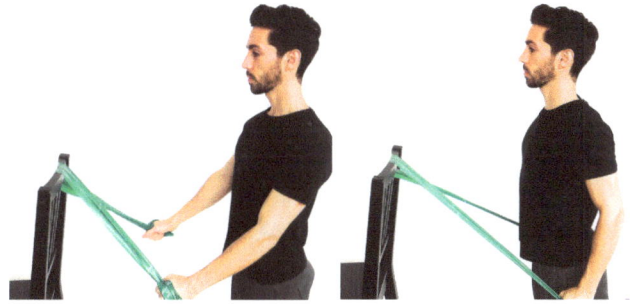

Loop a resistance band around a sturdy object. Hold either end, keep arms straight, step back and pull arms down and behind you.

Hold your arms behind you for 3 seconds, then slowly return to the starting position. Perform 3 sets of 10 reps.

B-9

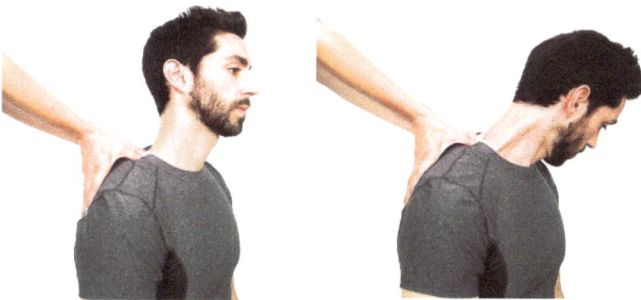

Have a friend push firmly just above the upper inner corner of your shoulder blade.

Slowly tilt your head down and away. Repeat 7 times on each side.

B-10

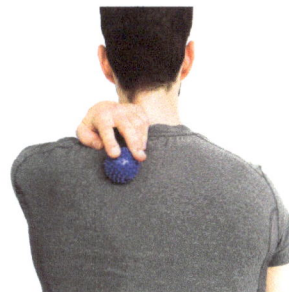

Lie on your back with the acuball mini placed where shown.

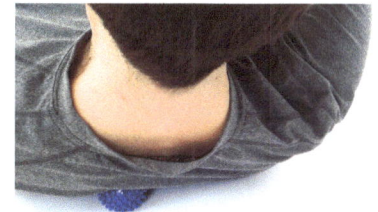

Use the other arm to lift the head up and to the opposite direction. Hold for 5 seconds. Repeat 3 times.

B-11

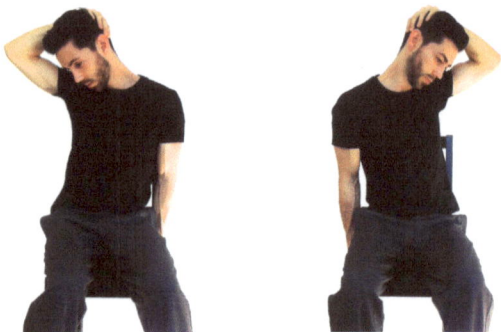

Sit on the palm of one hand so that you can't raise your shoulder. Use the other hand to pull your head gently down and to the opposite side.

Repeat on both sides. Hold the stretch for 30 seconds 3 times.

B - 12

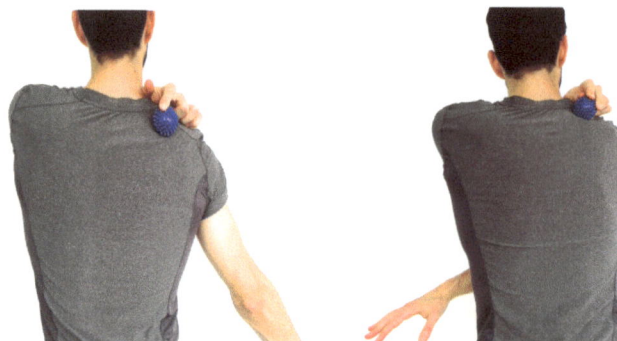

Place the acuball mini between you and the wall or the floor just above the upper ridge of the shoulder blade (spend a moment feeling for it). Once pressure is applied, move your arm slowly from your side across your body.

B - 13

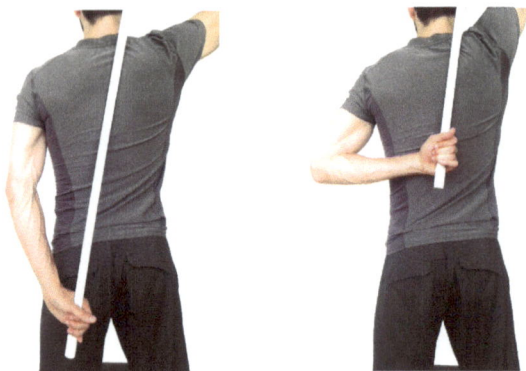

Hold a stick behind your back with one arm low and the other above your head.

Gently and slowly pull up with the higher arm to lift the lower. Hold at the end range for 3 seconds. Repeat 6 times.

B - 14

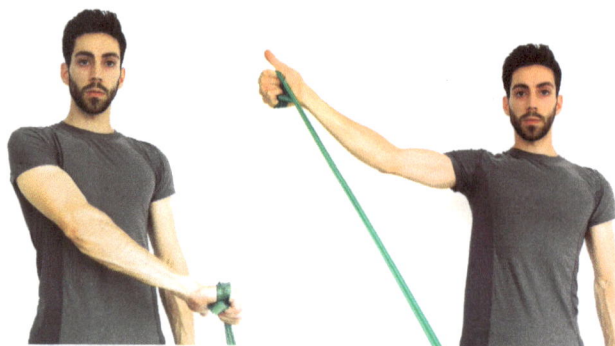

Attach a resistance band firmly to a sturdy object, stand next to it and hold the loose end with your thumb pointed down.

Start with your shoulder blade pulled back a little, then lift your arm slowly all the way up and rotate your thumb up. 3 sets of 10 reps.

B - 15

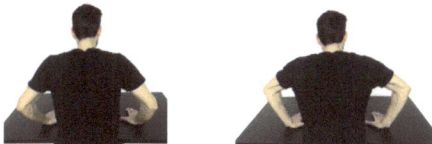

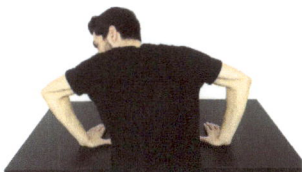

Place your hands on a waist-height table. Turn elbows out and bend them about 60 degrees.

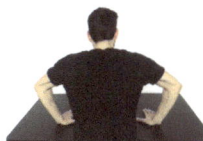

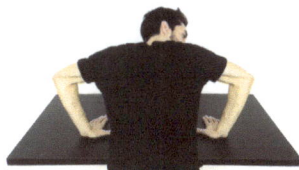

Keeping your elbows out and hands pointed in, reach your nose towards each elbow & hold for 5 seconds.

B - 16

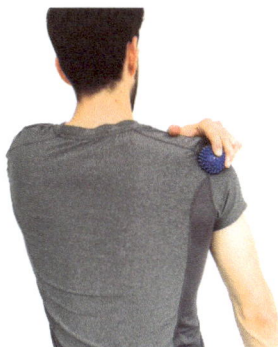

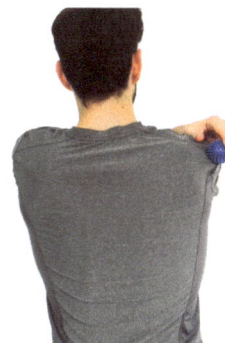

Place the ball just under the bony part of the back of your shoulder. Lean into it against a wall.

While leaning into the ball, slowly move your arm from your side all the way across your body and reach to the opposite side. Repeat 6 times.

B - 17

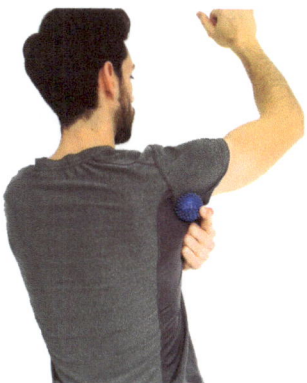

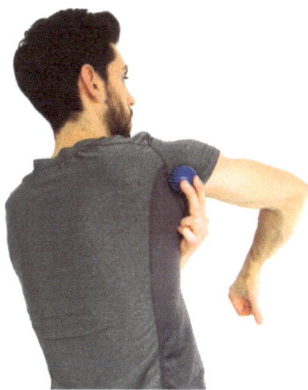

Lift your arm up, place the ball on the 'roof' of the back of your armpit and lean against a wall. Roll around until you find a tender point.

Holding the pressure against the wall, rotate your hand all the way down while keeping your elbow in place. Rotate up & down several times.

B - 18

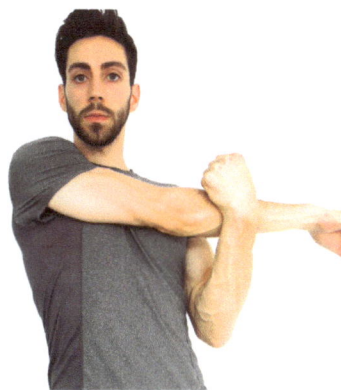

Pull your straight arm closer into your body with your other arm. Bend forward and twist slightly into the stretch to intensify.

B - 19

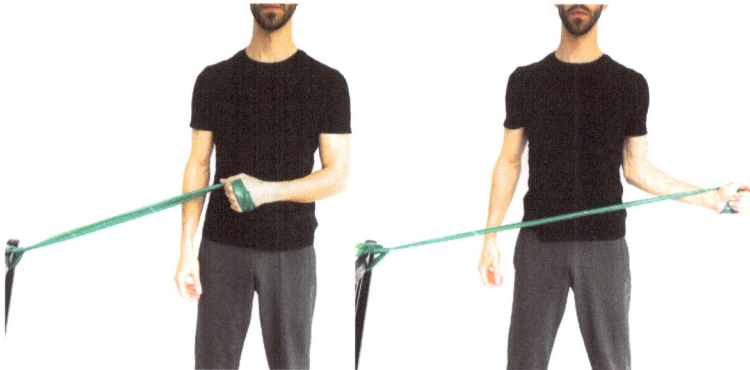

Attach one end of a resistance band to a sturdy object and wrap the other end around your hand. Stand as shown with the band at waist level.

Keeping your elbow still & tucked in, rotate your arm to pull the band slowly out & back in. Keep shoulder blades back. Do 3 sets of 10.

B - 20

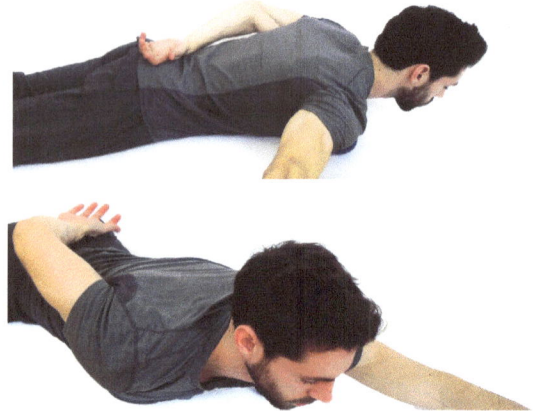

Place a ball just under your collarbone and lie on it face down. Stick your arm out to the side & begin by dropping your shoulder further to the ground.

Slowly move your arm up above your head and back down. This one takes a little finesse. Repeat 6 times.

B - 21

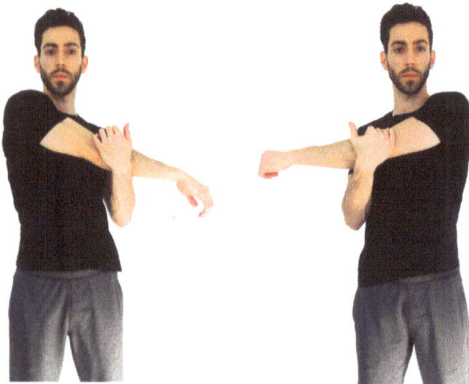

Pull your arm across your body.

Let your shoulder blade slide all the way forward while you stretch until you feel the pull in your midback.

B - 22

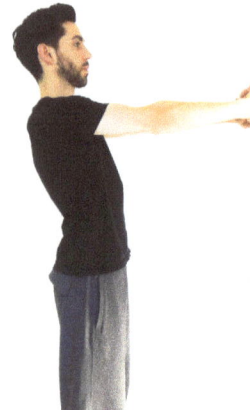

Interlock your fingers, keep your elbows straight and hands up at shoulder height. Start rotating your shoulder blades in big slow circles while keeping your hands where they are. Repeat 20 times.

B - 23

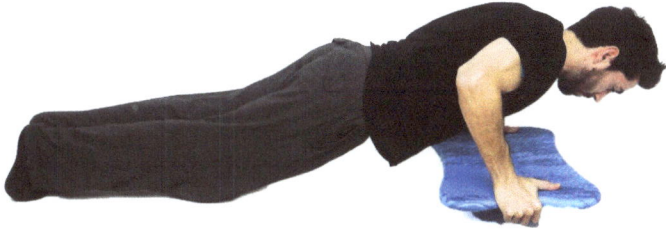

Perform pushups on a wobble board. Each rep should be done very slowly, controlled & with shoulder blades held together.

B - 24

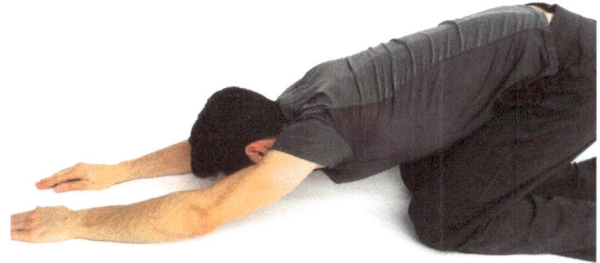

Lean forward on your knees with your arms stretched out above your head. Keep your back straight & bend in the hips.

Inch your hands forward as you breathe deeply. Feel the pull from your neck and shoulders, through your midback & low back.

B - 25

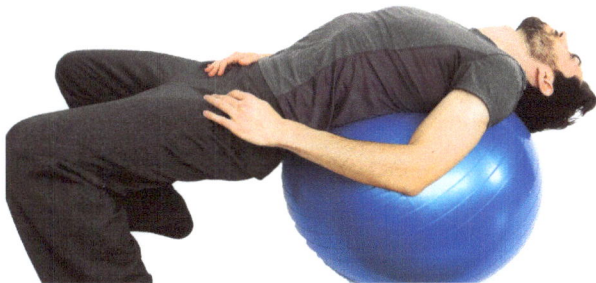

Carefully slide from sitting on a yoga ball to a lying position. Slowly relax your back to bend backwards with the contour of the ball. Hold the position for no more than a minute.

B - 26

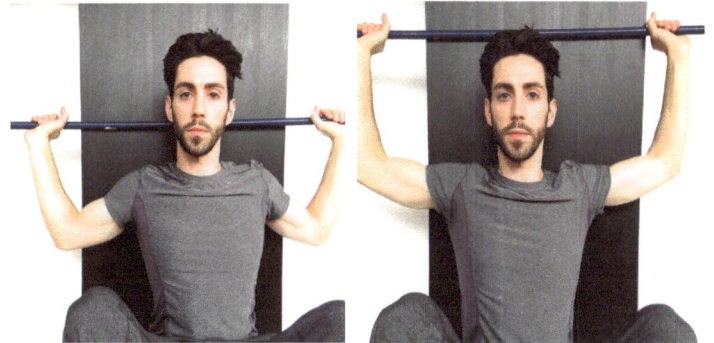

Sit with your back & shoulders against a wall. Holding a stick behind your head, slowly slide the stick up & down against the wall.

Slide up & down 20 times slowly, focusing on quality movement. Do 2-3 sets.

B - 27

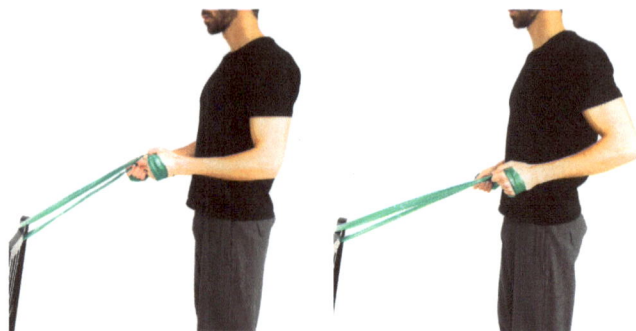

Hold both ends of a resistance band looped around a sturdy object at waist level. Start with your arms to your side & elbows bent to 90 degrees.

Pull your arms back, squeezing your shoulder blades together & return them slowly. Do 3 sets of 12 reps.

B - 28

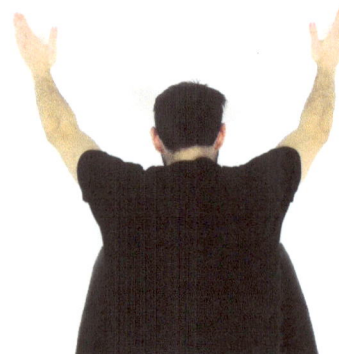

Pull your shoulder blades together and down. Holding your shoulder blades in place, slowly raise your arms straight up with thumbs up. Then slowly lower without letting your shoulder blades drop. Do 3 sets of 10.

B - 29

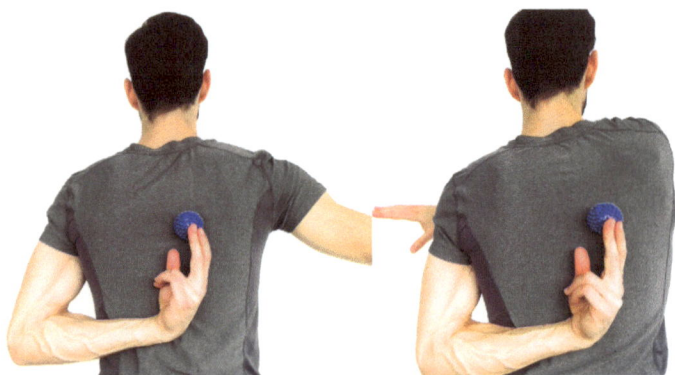

Place a ball in the space between your spine & shoulder blades in your mid back. Lean up against a wall or lie on your back.

Pushing your weight into the ball, start with your arm out to the side and slowly move it across your body, reaching for the opposite shoulder. Repeat 6 times.

B - 30

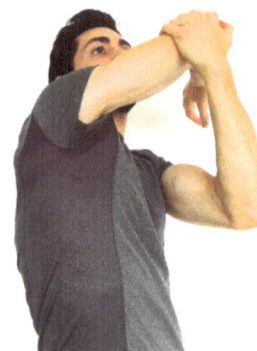

Bend your elbow and lift your arm so that your elbow is at the height of your nose. Lower your hand below your elbow. Use the other hand to pull the elbow gently towards the opposite shoulder.

B - 31

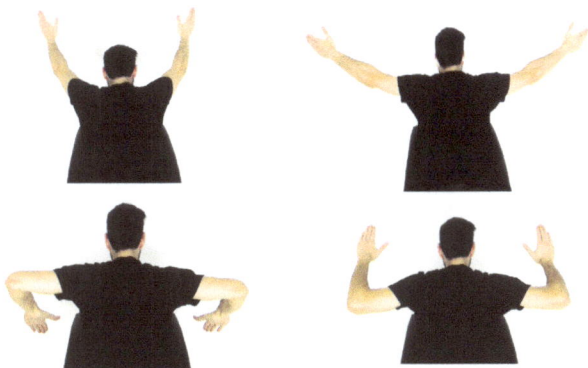

Lie on a bench face down. Pull your shoulder blades together and down. Hold blades together while you slowly bring your arms up into an 'I' position.

Start again, this time bringing arms up and out into a 'Y' position with thumbs up. Then into a 'T' position, first raising elbows then rotating arms so hands come up. Do 10 reps of each.

B - 32

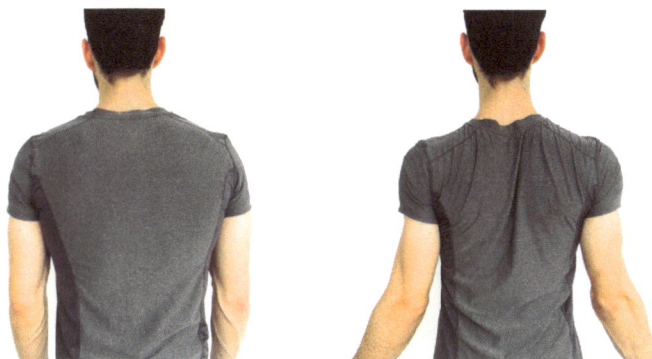

Lift your shoulder blades up & roll your shoulders back.

Rotate your palms to face forward, squeeze your shoulder blades firmly together, then pull them all the way down. Repeat 30 times.

B - 33

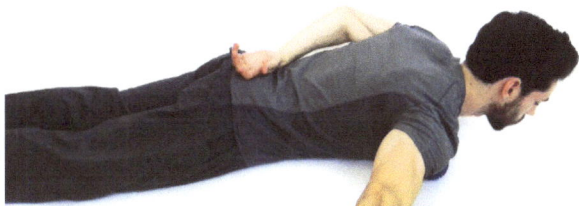

Lying on your stomach, put a ball on a tender area in the upper outer quadrant of your breast area. With your arm out to the side, slowly move your arm up & down off the ground while moving it progressively higher towards your head.

B - 34

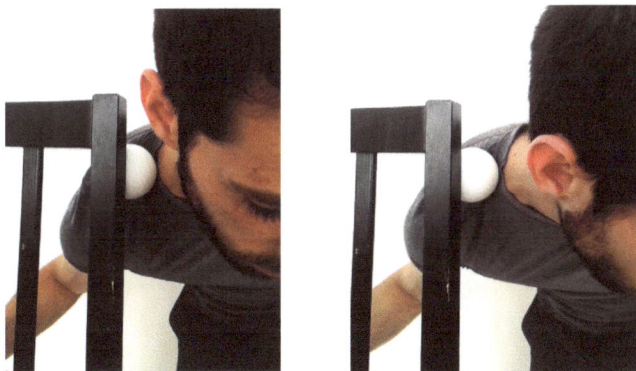

Find a doorway. Bend your torso 90 dregrees, leaning into the door frame. Place a ball at the base of your trapezius - roughy in line with your ear & on a tender spot.

Lean into the ball with your body. Then slowly tilt your head away from the shoulder while maintaining pressure. Repeat 6 times.

C - 1

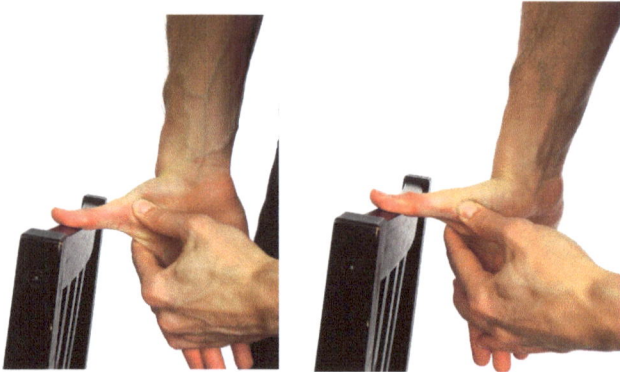

Place your thumb on the edge of a surface. Push into a tender spot firmly with your other thumb.

Move your arm down to further extend your thumb & stretch the muscle that you're pushing in on. Repeat 6 times.

C - 2

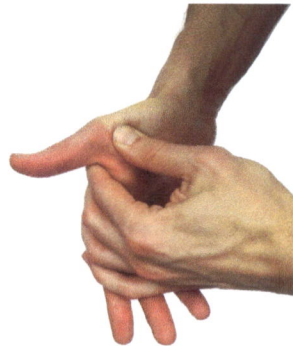

Push into a tight or tender spot at the base of your thumb. Hold the pressure while you slowly move along the length of the tight muscle to stretch it.

C - 3

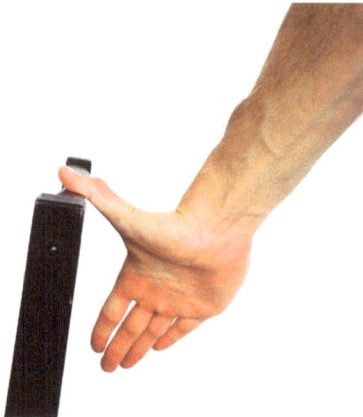

Stretch the thumb muscles by moving your arm down with your thumb on the edge of a surface.

C - 4

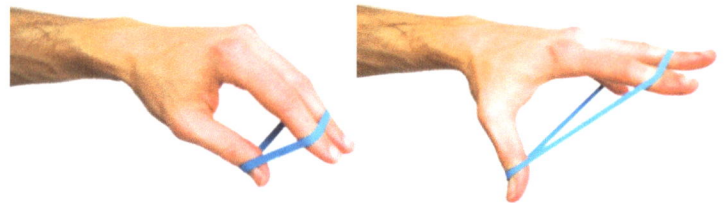

Start with a neutral wrist and fingers close together.

Spread all fingers fully out. Hold for a second before closing the fingers. Do 2 sets of 10 reps.

C-5

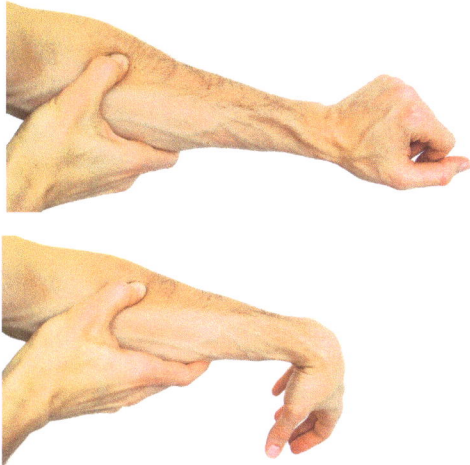

Push firmly into a tender point on the muscle on the thumb side of the back of your forearm, closer to the elbow.

Hold firm pressure while you bend the wrist slowly all the way down. Repeat 8 times.

C-6

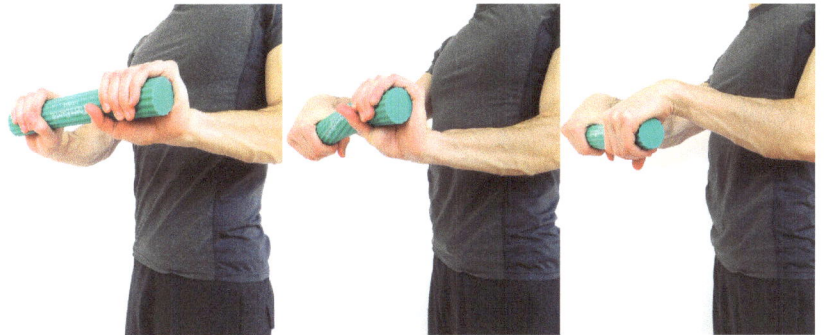

Grib the flexbar with both hands, begin with both wrists up.

If working your right hand, begin by twisting only the left hand down. Hold the position with the other hand.

Lower the right wrist very slowly to un-twist the flexbar. Do 3 sets of 10.

C-7

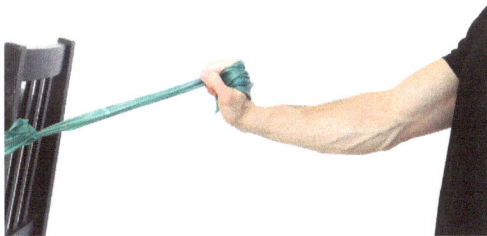

Secure a resistance band around a sturdy object and around your hand. Start with your wrist back, then move your arms back to create tension.

Slowly let your wrist bend down against the resistance. Then return to the starting position without resistance. Do 3 sets of 10.

C-8

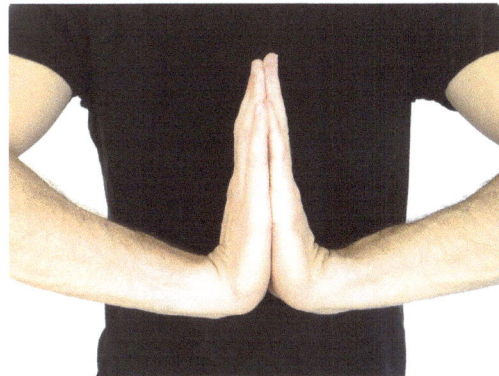

Place your palms together with fingers pointed up. Hold for 30 seconds. Feel the stretch in the underside of your forearms.

C - 9

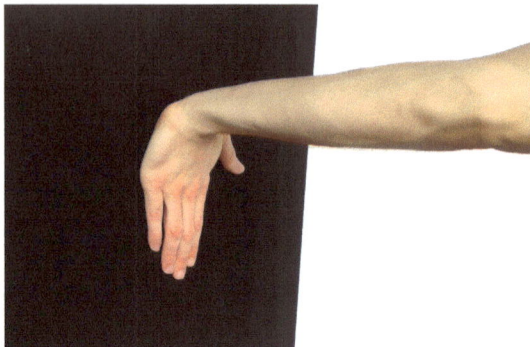

With fingers pointed down and elbow straight, push your palm into a wall at waist height. Hold for 30 seconds. Repeat 2 or 3 times.

C - 10

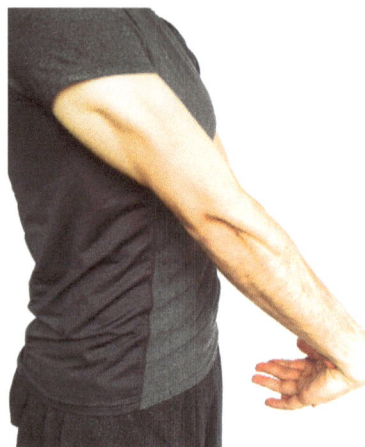

Stretch the upper forearm muscles by pulling your hand down while keeping your elbow straight. Your palm should be facing your face. Hold for 20 seconds.

C - 11

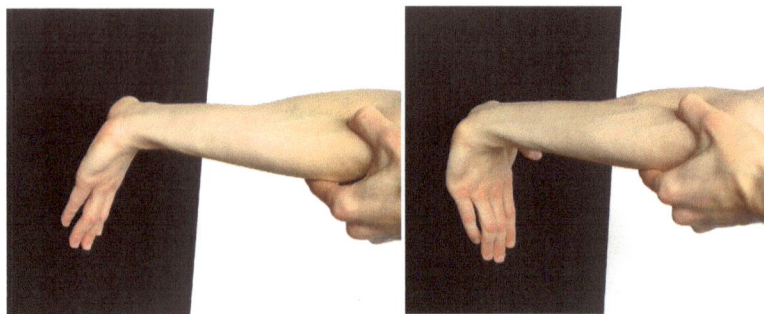

Find and push into a tender point in your forearm muscles. With elbow straight and fingers pointed down, move your palm closer to the wall.

Continue to push into the muscle along its length. Repeat 6 times.

C - 12

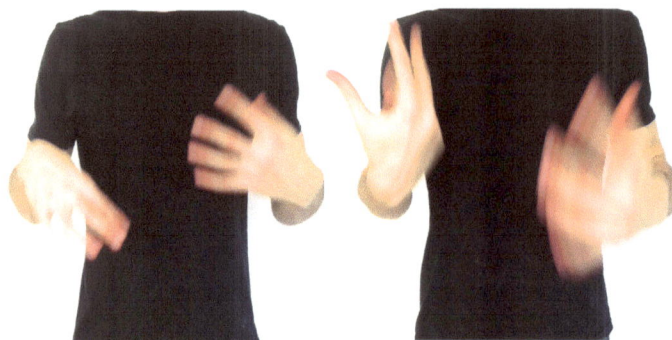

Shake shake shake

Gently shake the wrists in all directions. Helping to relax some of the muscles, repeat when needed.

C - 13

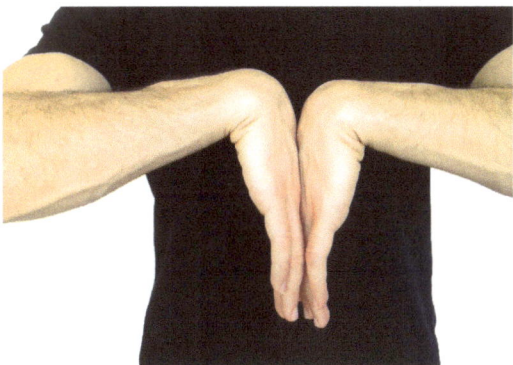

With fingers pointed down and palms turned out, gently push the top of the wrists together. Hold for 15 seconds.

C - 14

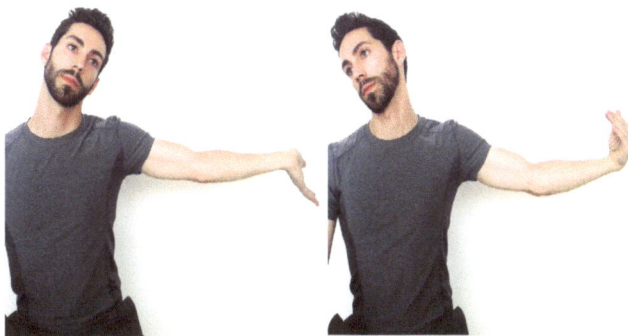

Hold your arm straight out to your side with palm up. Tilt your head down towards that side while simultaneously tilting the wrist down.

'Floss' the nerve by alternating into the opposite position- tilting your wrist up and the head to the opposite direction simultaneously. Repeat 12 times.

C - 15

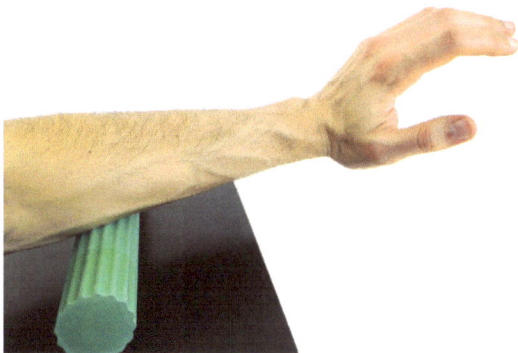

Roll the tense forearm muscles on a flexbar. Tilt the wrist up and put more weight into it to intensify. Roll for a minute.

C - 16

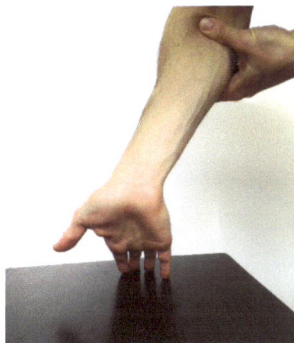

Pull the skin up and push firmly into a tender spot just south of the elbow.

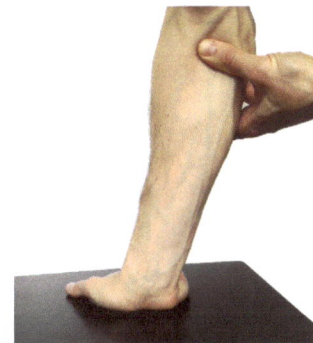

Hold the pressure while you lower the palm to be flat on the wall or table. Keep the elbow straight. Repeat 6 times.

C - 17

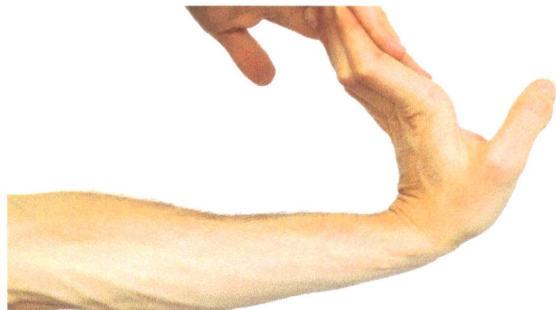

Keep your elbow straight and use the other hand to pull your hand and fingers up and back.

C - 18

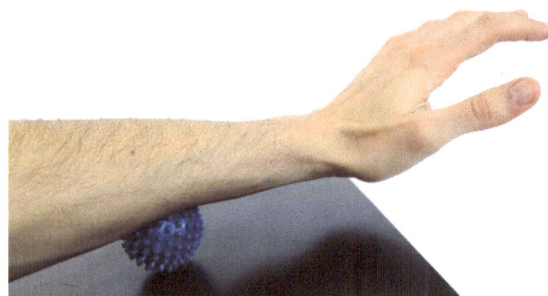

Put pressure on an acuball with your forearm. Slowly roll and push into tender areas. Lift wrist to intensify.

C - 19

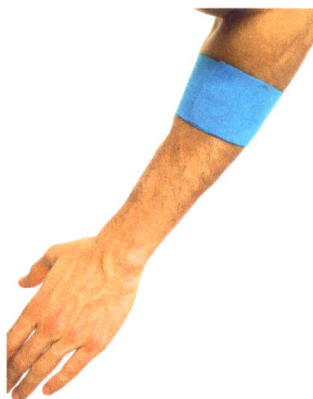

Apply kinesiology tape around the upper third of the forearm. Tape tension should be roughly 50%.

C - 20

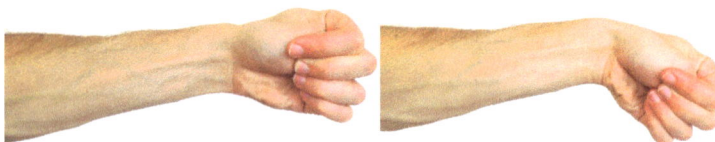

Tuck your thumb into your fist.

Bend the wrist all the way down in the direction of the pinky finger.

C - 21

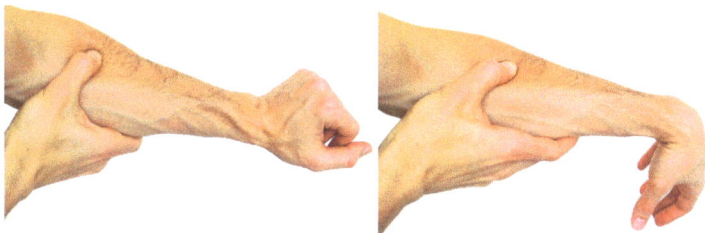

Find the tender spot & apply pressure on the back of the forearm just past the elbow.

Hold pressure while bending the wrist all the way down. Repeat 6 times.

C - 22

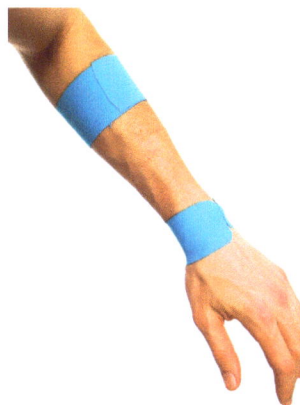

Apply kinesiology tape to the forearm and to the wrist with 40-50% tension.

C - 23

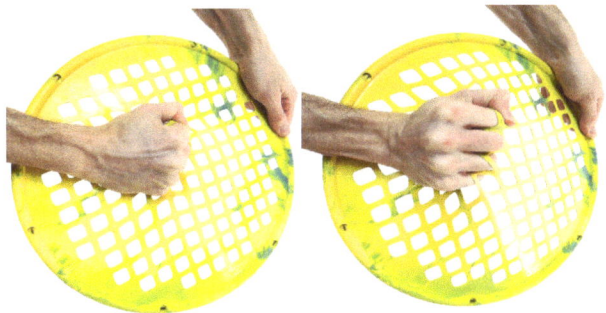

Grab the power web & pull your hand out & back.

Perform 2 sets of 10 slow reps.

C - 24

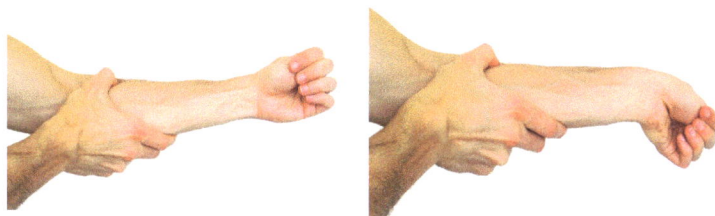

With your wrist turned out, push in at the apex (top) of the forearm, into the tender muscle bulk. Tuck your thumb.

Hold the pressure while you lower the wrist as far as you can. Repeat 6 times.

C - 25

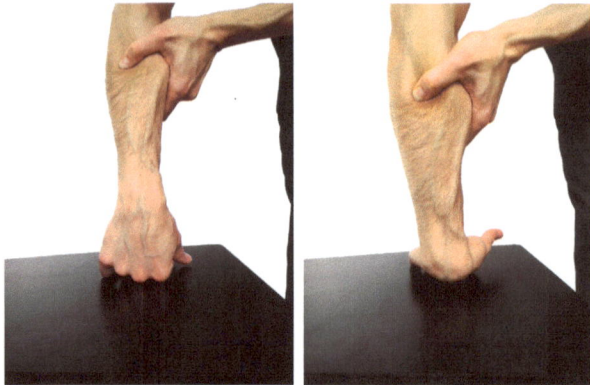

Line your fist up against a wall. Push into a tight spot on your forearm, closer to the elbow, on the pinky side.

Press firmly while you push your arm into the wall to bend the wrist down. Repeat 6 times.

C - 26

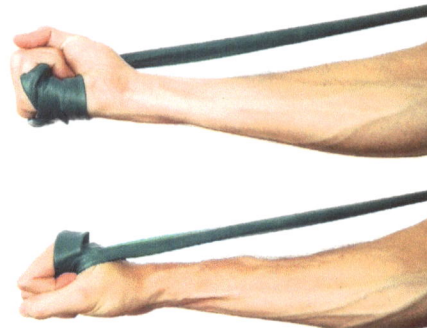

Wrap a resistance band around your hand and attach the other end to an object. Stand beside the object.

Slowly turn your hand in and down all the way against resistance. Do 3 sets of 6 reps.

C - 27

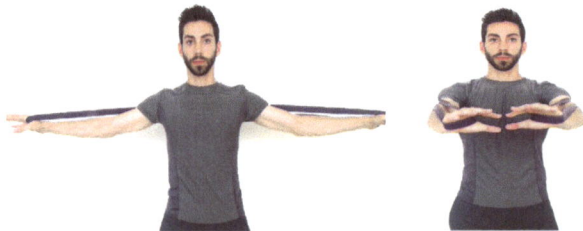

Pull a strong resistance band tight behind your shoulders.

Bring your arms slowly forward until they meet eachother. Do 20 slow reps.

C - 28

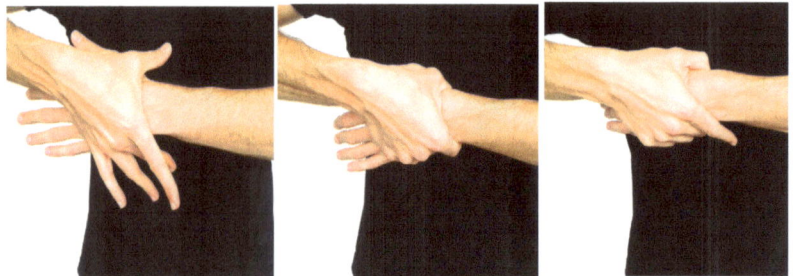

With a straight and neutral wrist, wrap your thumb and finger of the other hand tightly around the indents at the smallest point of your wrist. Grip firmly and evenly, keep the wrist neutral. Gently pull the wrist away from the arm. Hold for 1 second. Do it carefully and not more than 5 times.

C - 29

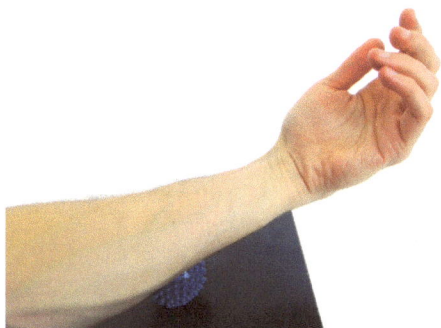

Roll the acuball along the tender points on the back of your forearm. Push in or bend wrist up to intensify. On particularly tight or tender spots, hold the pressure on that spot while you slowly bend the wrist up & down.

C - 30

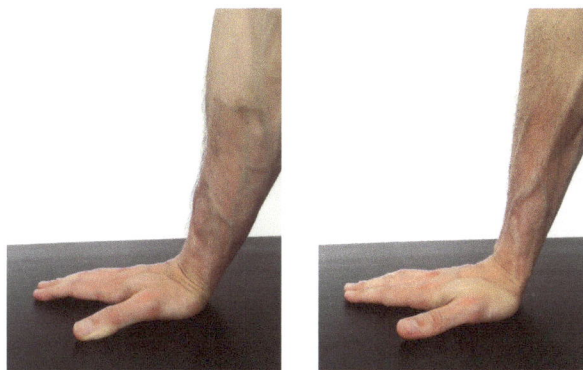

Place your palm flat on a surface with a bit of weight into it.

Without moving your hand, slowly rotate your arm all the way to one side and to the other. Repeat 5 times.

C - 31

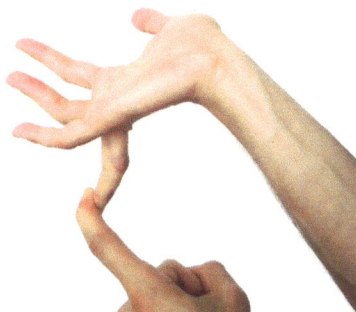

With the elbow straight and wrist bent back, pull each finger down towards the back of the forearm and hold for 10 seconds.

C - 32

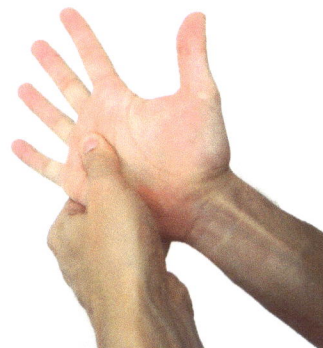

Open the hand and spread your fingers out wide. Start with your other thumb pushing firmly into the centre of your hand. Slowly & firmly push in and slide along the palm up towards the fingers. Continue until the tension is reduced.

C - 33

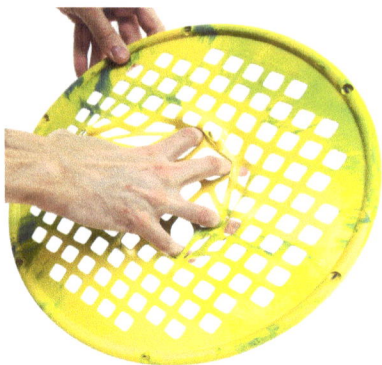

Place your fingers into the web close together. Spread your fingers & hold for 2 seconds 10 times.

C - 34

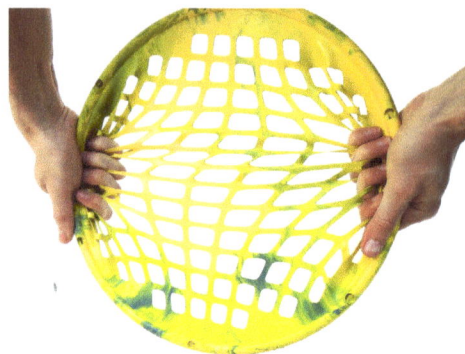

Grab both sides of the power web with tension. Release the tension extra slowly. Repeat 15 times.

C - 35

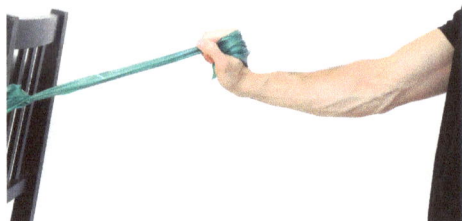

Attach one end of a resistance band to a sturdy object and the other around your hand. First tilt your wrist up, then move your arm away until it is moderately tense. Slowly lower your wrist against the tension. Do 3 sets of 10 reps.

C - 36

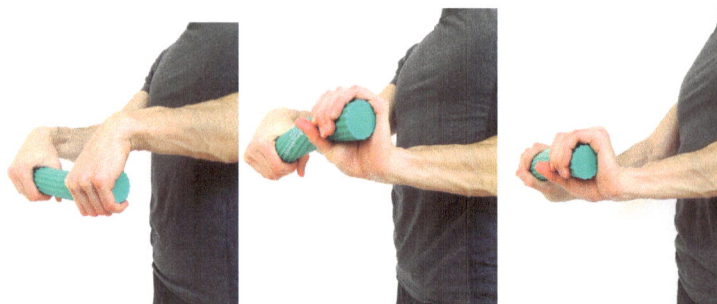

Grib the flexbar with both hands, begin with both wrists down.

If working your right hand, begin by twisting only the left hand up. Hold the position with the other hand.

Raise the right wrist very slowly to un-twist the flexbar. Do 3 sets of 10.

C - 37

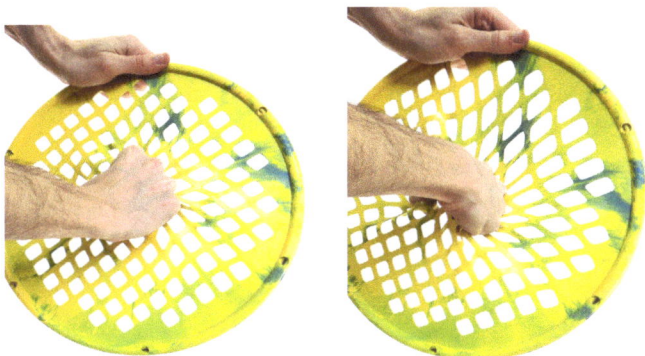

Grab the power web and make a fist.

Tilt your wrist down, hold for 1 seconds & slowly release. Do 2 sets of 10 reps.

C - 38

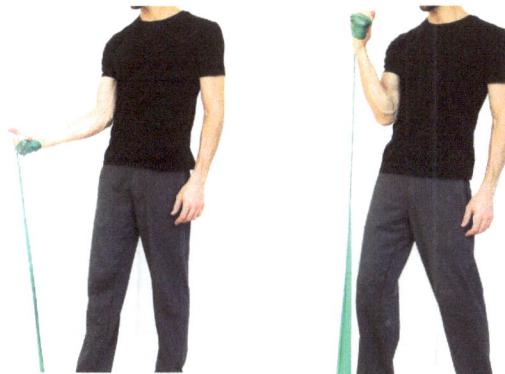

Wrap one end of a resistance band around your foot securely. Hold the band at mid-thigh level, stand straight up, keep your elbow right against your body next to your hip. Slowly bend your elbow, pulling the band up. 3 seconds up, 3 seconds down.

C - 39

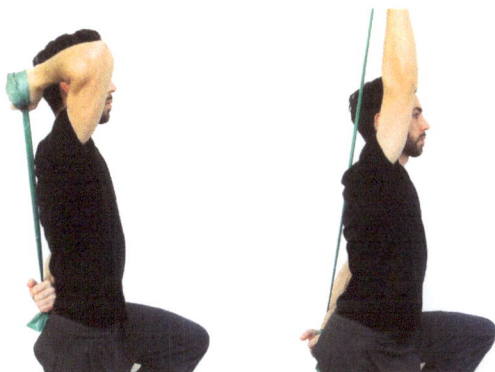

Hold one end of a resistance band behind your low back. With the other hand, hold the band behind your head, with your elbow beside your head and slowly straighten your arm. Increase or decrease the tension using your non-active hand. Do 2 sets of 10 reps with each arm.

C - 40

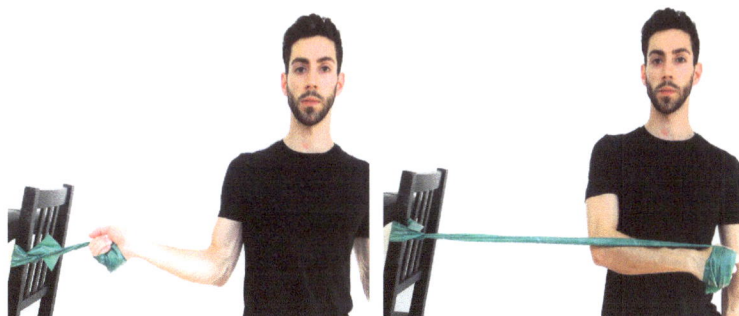

Stand with the band attached to an immovable object to the same side of you as the target shoulder. Keep your elbow tucked in while slowly pulling the band across your body. 3 seconds in, 3 seconds back out.

C - 41

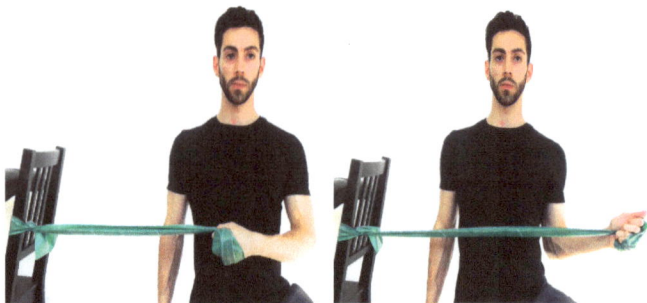

Attach a band to something that won't move. Stand with the object beside you to the opposite side of the working shoulder. Keep your elbow against your torso while slowly pulling the band all the way out and slowly back. 3 seconds out, 3 seconds back

C - 42

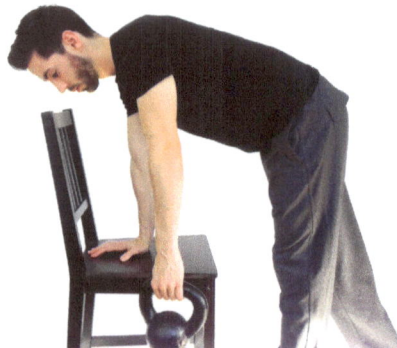

Hold any object that weighs a few pounds. Lean forward, supporting yourself with your other arm. Let the weighted arm hang and just dangle, focus on letting the shoulder muscles relax. Gently oscillate the weight in small circles. Continue to focus on relaxing the upper arm muscles. 2 minutes.

C - 43

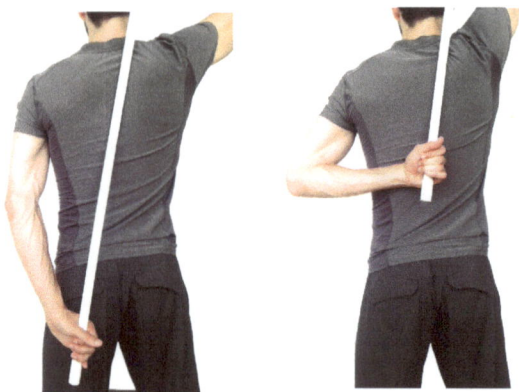

Hold a broomstick with one hand behind your low back and the other above your head. Slowly raise the stick, gently using your upper arm to stretch the lower and then lower the stick, pulling gently down with the lower hand to stretch the upper shoulder. Repeat 10 times for each arm.

C - 44

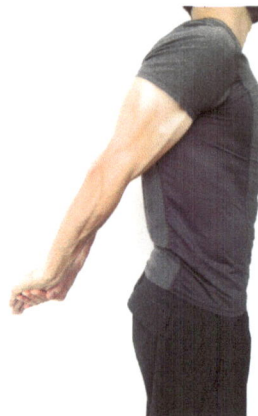

Clasp hands together behind your back and raise your hands slowly as high as you can comfortably.

C - 45

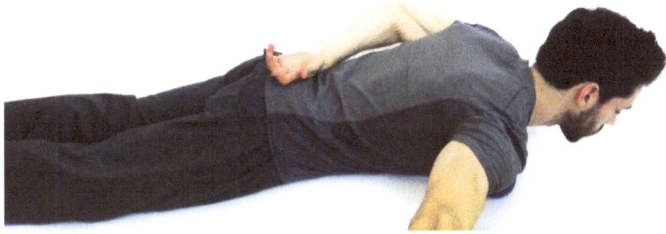

Place the acuball between your chest and shoulder, then let your weight apply pressure into the ball. Hold for 30 seconds. Lying face down on the ground or up against a wall.

C - 46

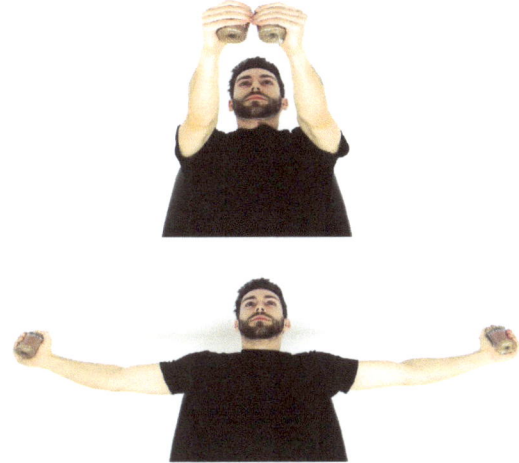

Lying on a bench, hold weights up in front of you with straight arms and slowly lower arms down to your side. 3 seconds on the way down, 3 seconds up.

C - 47

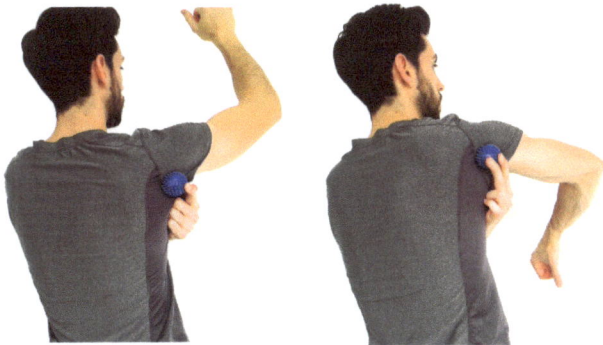

Place the acuball about 2 inches in from the back of your armpit. Push it up against a wall. Once on a tense spot, keep your elbow up and slowly rotate your hand down and up.

C - 48

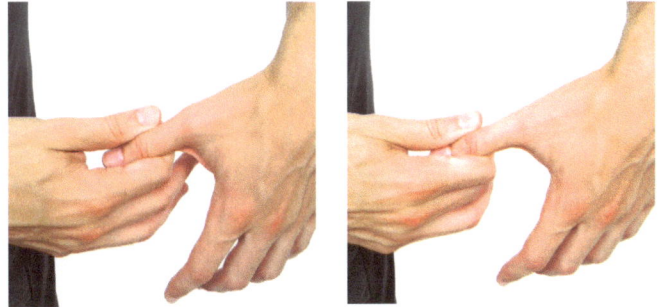

Grasp your thumb firmly and pull gently away from the hand, hold for 2 seconds then release.

C - 49

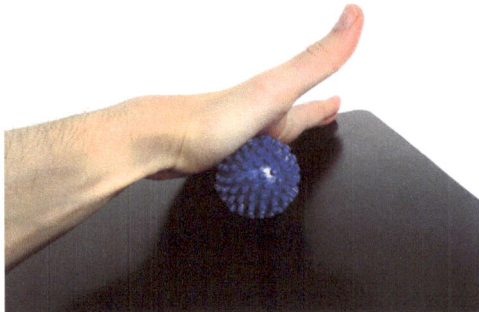

Roll the ball firmly all around the underside of your lower thumb.

C - 50

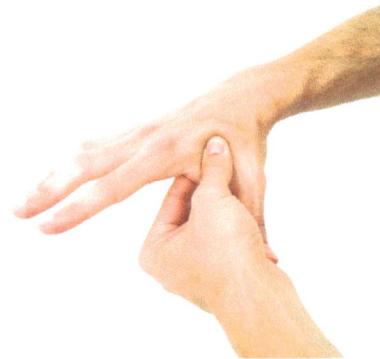

Squeeze the bulk of tissue between your first finger and thumb firmly for 30 seconds.

C - 51

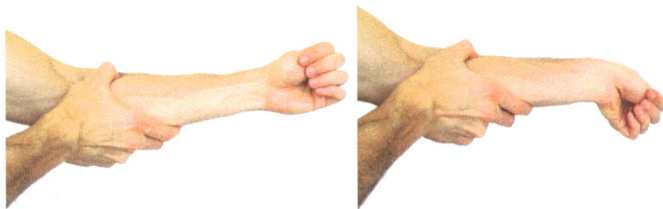

Find the most tender point of the muscle near the elbow crease.

Use your thumb to hold firm pressure on the point while tilting your wrist up & down - thumb to the roof and pinky to the floor.

C - 52

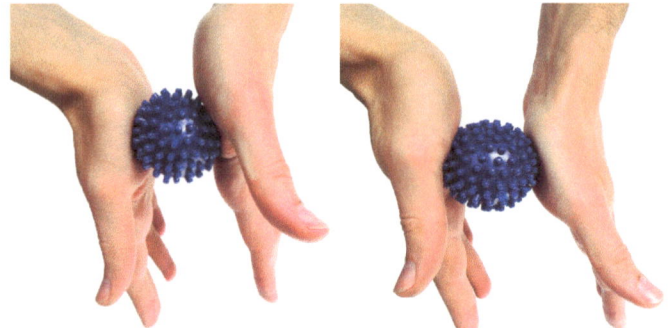

Squeeze the acuball between the lower inner part of both thumbs.

Roll it around and then hold it in the tender spots for 10-20 seconds.

C - 53

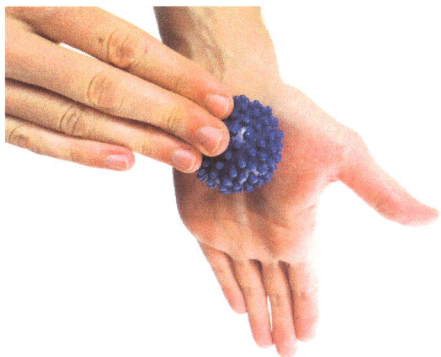

With moderate pressure, roll the ball in the grooves between the long bones in your hand that correspond with each finger. Try rolling on both the palm side and the back side of your hand.

C - 54

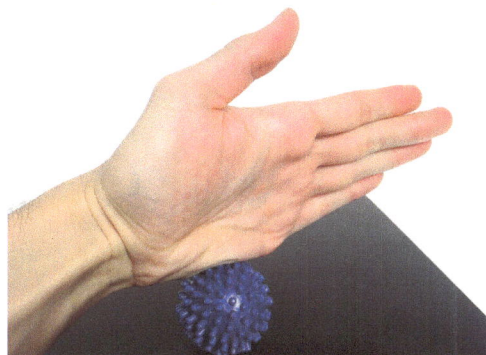

Roll the acuball firmly and slowly along the edge of your hand on the side of your pinky finger. Try with your pinky finger a little forward and a little backward.

C - 55

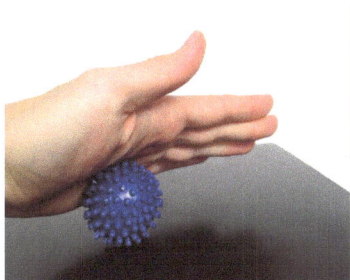

Roll the ball slowly around the palm of your hand with moderate pressure.

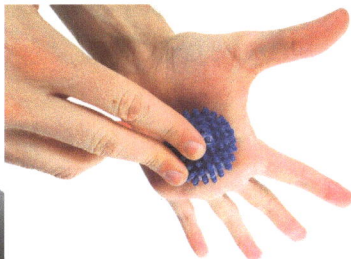

First roll with your hand relaxed and then with your fingers stretched back and palm spread.

C - 56

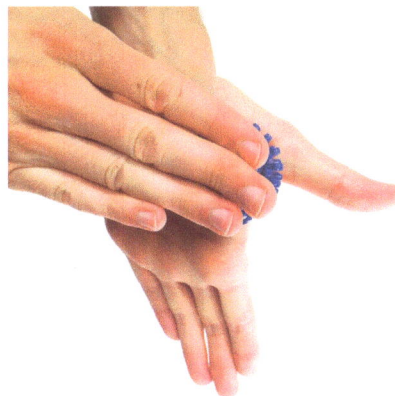

Push the base of your thumb into the ball until you feel a tense/tender spot. Maintain pressure while you slowly move your thumb in and out.

D - 1

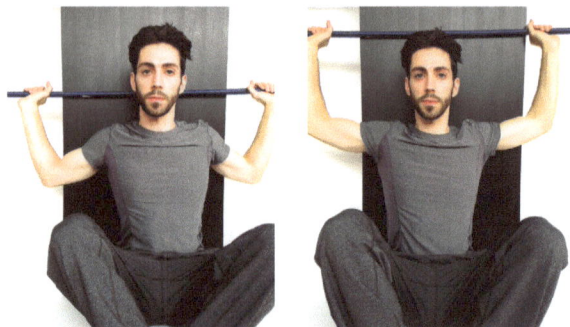

Sit with your back against a wall. Hold a broomstick (or equivalent) against the wall just above your head.

Hands should line up with shoulders. Slowly raise the stick up and back down. Do 3 sets of 8.

D - 2

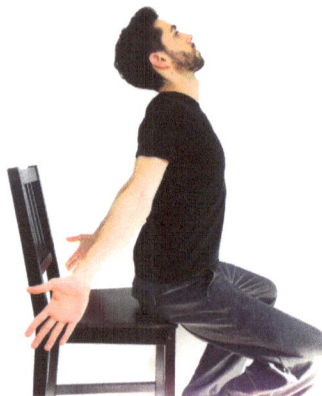

Sit on the edge of a chair with your knees spread wider than your hips and toes pointed slightly outward. Tuck your chin, take a deep breath and as you breath out actively, turn your palms out, your arms back and your chest forward. Hold your chest out for 5 seconds. Repeat 3 times.

D - 3

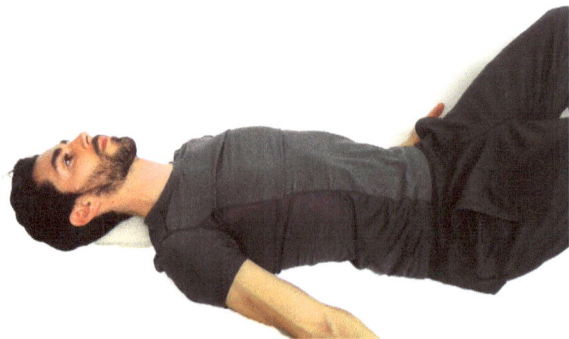

Roll a towel so that it's about as wide as your fist. Lie down with it lengthwise along your spine. Arms out to the side. Breathe deeply and relax.

D - 4

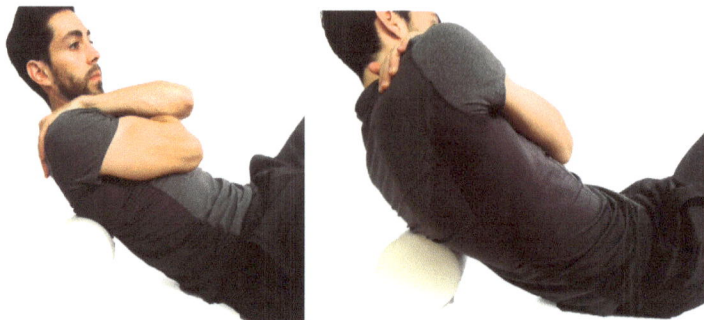

Give yourself a hug, roll slowly a few inches up and down the mid and upper back with the foam roller just off to either side. Be careful and do this slowly.

D-5

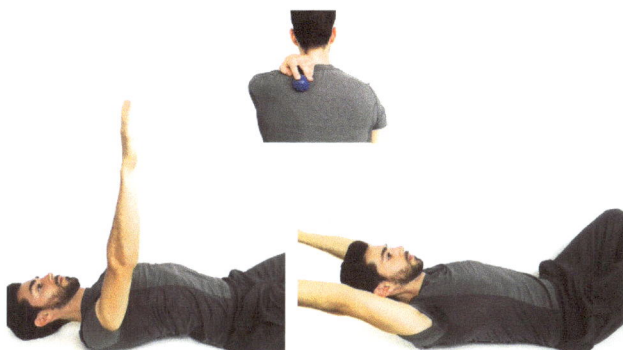

Place the acuball between the spine and shoulder blade.

Roll around a little to find a tight/tender spot. Slowly raise arm all the way up and back down.

D-6

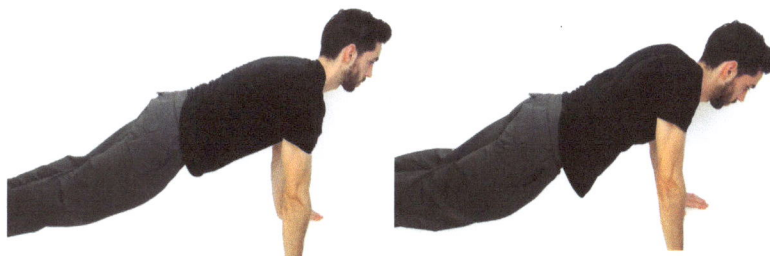

Begin in a pushup position. Keeping elbows fully straight, lower your torso down at the shoulder.

Hold the lowered position for 1 second and then push back up. Movement should be slow and controlled. Repeat 3 sets of 15.

D-7

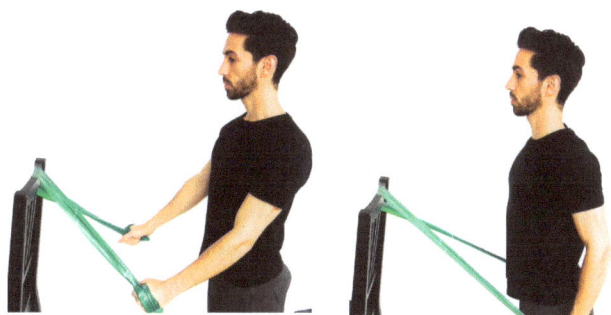

Holding both ends of a resistance band secured to a solid object, keep the arms straight and the shoulder blades together.

Pull your arms slowly all the way back and down. Repeat 3 sets of 15.

E-1

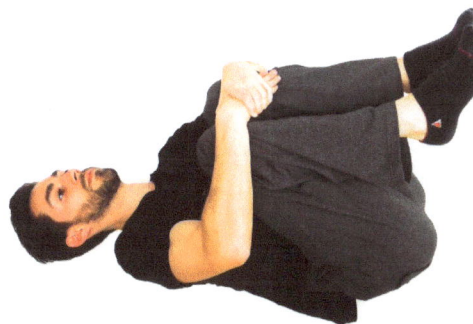

Lying on your back, bend both knees and bring your legs up towards your chest. Clasp your hands around your knees. Hold for 30 seconds.

E - 2

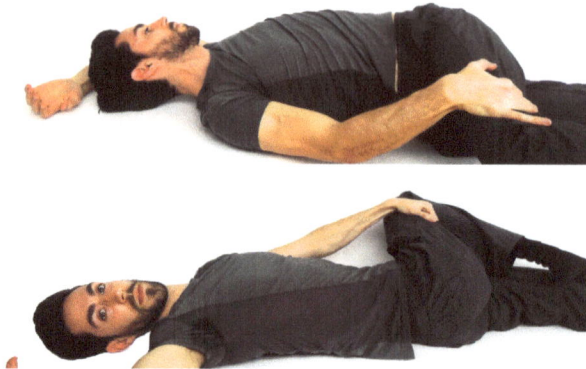

Lying on your back, bring one leg across your body until the inside of your knee touches the ground.

Extend your opposite arm out and keep the shoulder on the ground. Hold for 30 seconds on each side.

E - 3

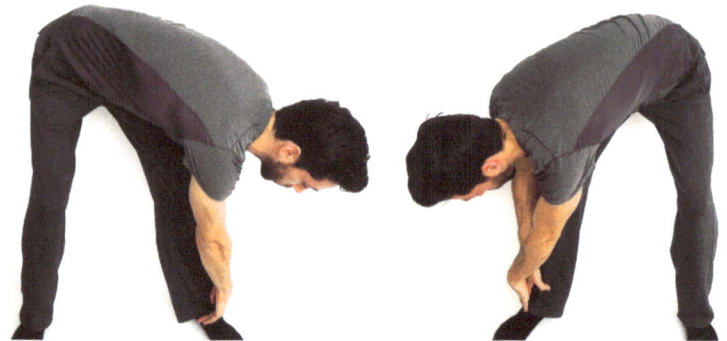

Standing with knees straight and legs a bit wider than shoulder width apart, bring your torso down towards one leg. Pull your torso towards one ankle at a time.

E - 4

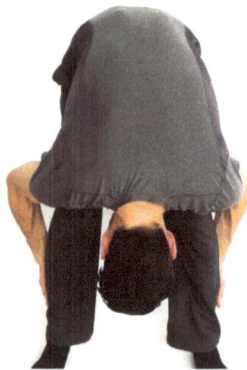

Keeping your legs straight, allow your torso to fold down all the way forward. Then gently grab the back of your legs and pull your body closer together.

OR

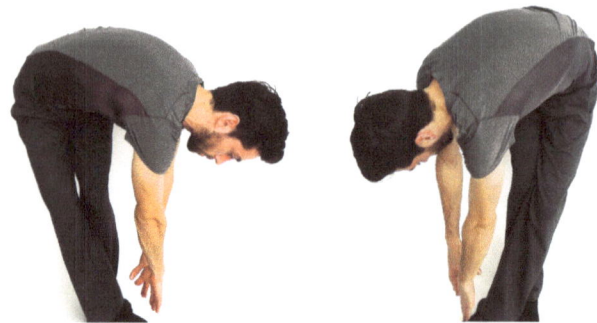

Stand with legs a couple feet apart and knees straight. Tilt as far as you can to one side, then slowly let your torso fold down towards the leg of that side.

E - 5

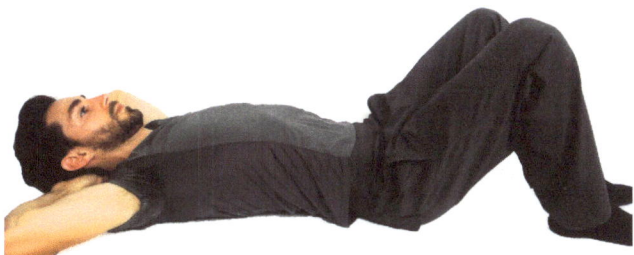

Lying on your back with legs straight or knees bent slightly. Roll your pelvis all the way backwards and forwards. Move slowly and focus on moving only your pelvis. 30 slow repetitions.

E - 6

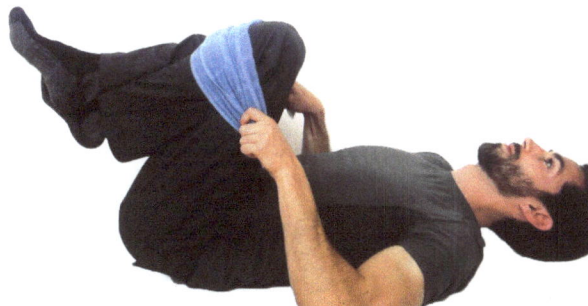

Lying on your back, hold either end of a towel strung around bent knees.

Use the towel to gently roll your knees from side to side.

E - 7

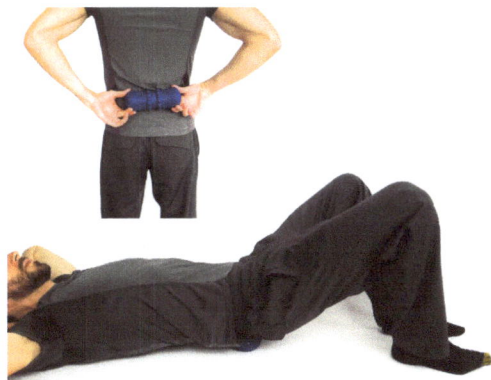

Lying on your back, place an acuball or acuback in the small of your low back, aligned carefully with the centre of your spine. If you feel pressure, breathe into it and relax. Slowly and gently roll up and down over the ball.

E - 8

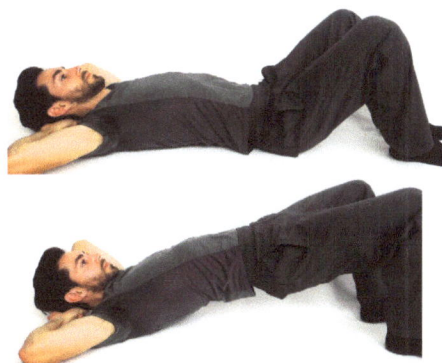

Lying on your back, bend your knees and plant your feet.

Slowly lift your bottom off the ground, squeeze and hold for 2 seconds and then relax. Repeat 30 times.

E - 9

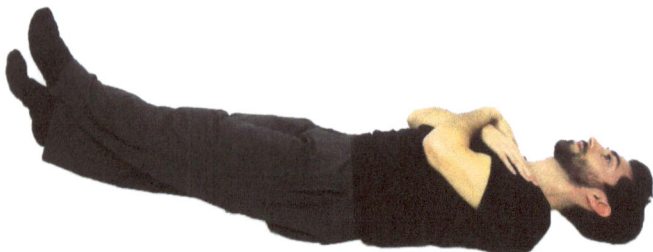

Lying on your back, lift both legs several inches off the ground. Cross your legs at the ankles, push up with the lower leg and push down with the upper leg. Hold for 10 seconds.

E - 10

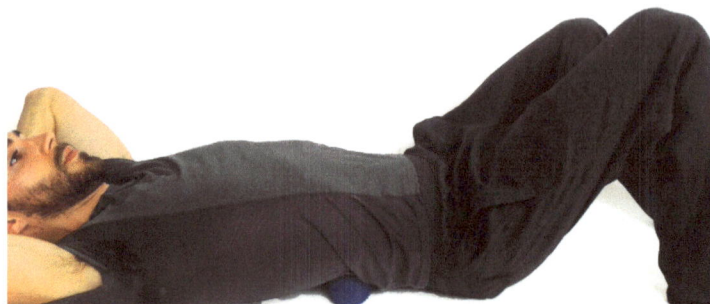

Be patient with this one, it may take a while to get it right. Lying flat on your back, wedge a warm acuball into your flank (side of torso, between ribs and pelvis). Slowly edge your body further overtop of the ball bit by bit until you feel great pressure or tenderness. Keep the ball on the tender spot and try to relax, take deep long breaths.

E - 11

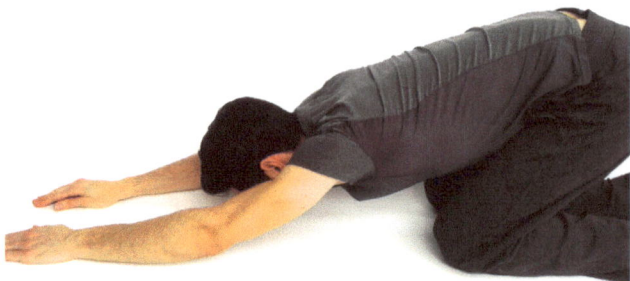

Start in a kneeling position. Sink down until you're sitting on your feet. Reach as far forward as you can with straight arms, then slowly sink your torso down to the ground. Hold for 45 seconds.

E - 12

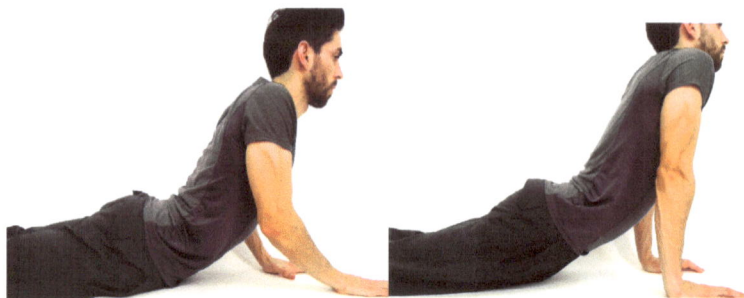

Lying on your stomach, use your hands to slowly lift your upper body up.

Keep your lower half relaxed. Once your elbows are straight, hold the pose for 20 seconds.

E - 13

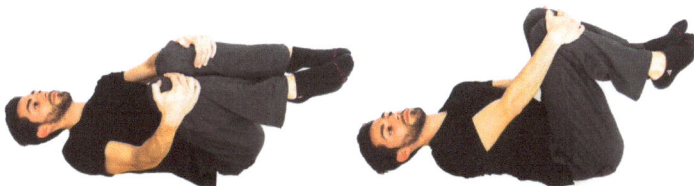

Lying on your back on a yoga mat, hold both knees bent and together.

Slowly start moving your knees as a unit in a small circle.

E - 14

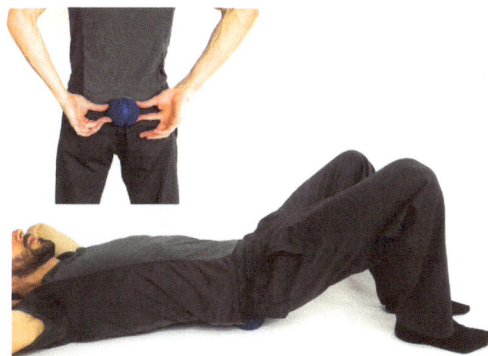

Align the heated acuball so that the ridge is vertical along the very middle of your tailbone. Lie on your back with bent knees and allow your weight to bear down on the ball and relax your muscles. Continue to breathe and relax with the tailbone on the ball for 2-5 minutes. You can substitute the ball for a roll of toilet paper.

E - 15

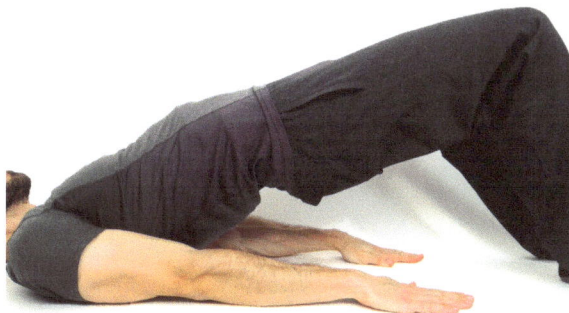

Lying on your back with arms straight to the side, plant both feet on the ground and lift your pelvis slowly as high as you can. Hold for 5 seconds. Repeat 10 times.

E - 16

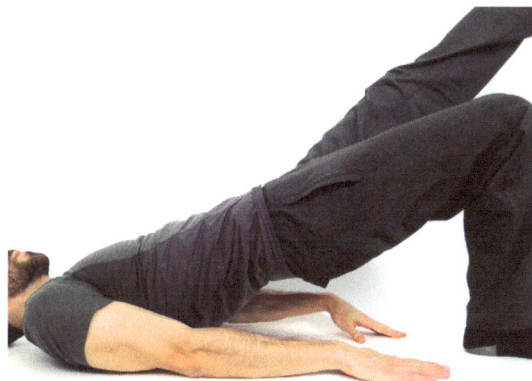

Lying on your back with arms straight to your side, lift one leg a foot off the floor and point it straight ahead.

Bend the other knee and lift your pelvis off the floor and hold for 5 seconds before slowly lowering back down.

E - 17

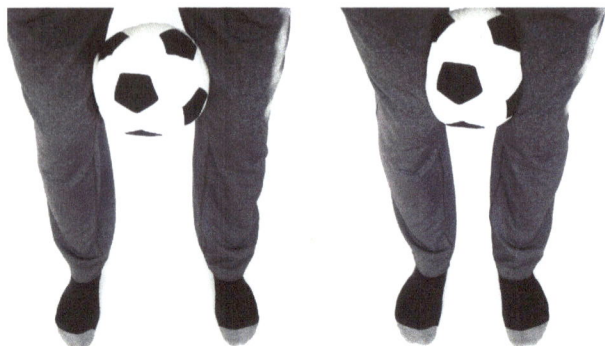

Standing or sitting with your legs together and straight, squeeze your legs together as firmly as you can and hold for 5 seconds.

Place towel or object between knees for added comfort. Repeat 30 times.

E - 18

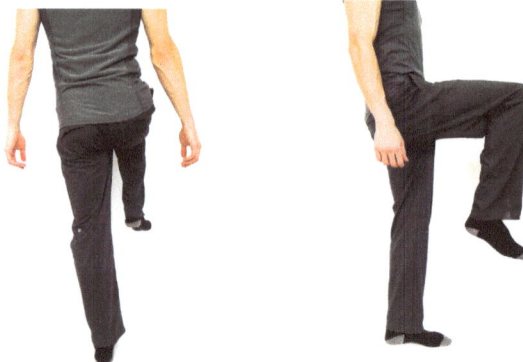

Standing with legs shoulder width apart, raise one leg until hip & knee are at 90 degrees.

Hold for 2 seconds then lower. Maintain a level pelvis throughout the whole movement. Do 20 reps for each leg.

E - 19

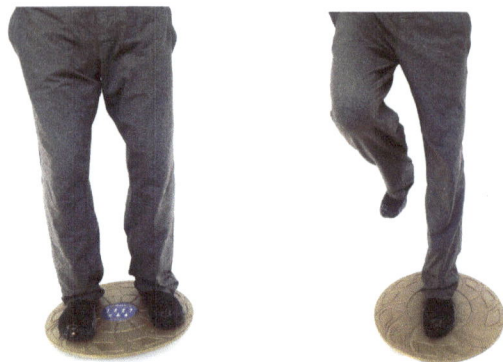

Stand and balance on a wobble board. Work towards standing without tipping for several minutes.

Then stand on the wobble board with one leg and do the same.

F - 1

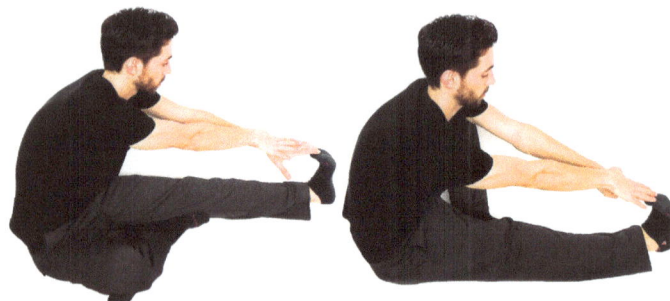

Sit with one knee bent and the other leg straight. Reach for the foot of your straight leg with both hands.

Hold the stretch for 30 seconds. Repeat twice.

F-2

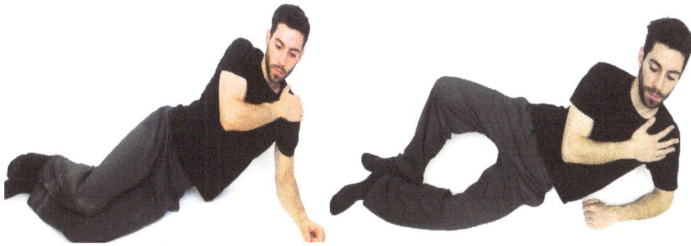

Lying on your side with knees bent and ankles together, slowly lift your top knee all the way up and back down.

Hold your knee up and squeeze your gluteal muscle for 3 seconds for each rep. Do 3 sets of 10 reps. Add a resistance band for more intensity.

F-3

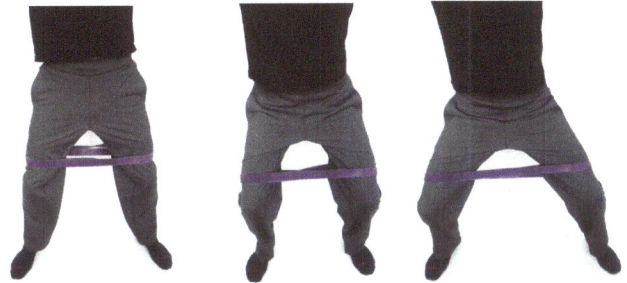

With a thick resistance band around your thighs above your knees, start in a half squat position (see F-4 details for form) and take 5 slow, wide side steps.

Keep your squat form and stay level (do not bob up & down). Walk ten lengths in each direction and then repeat.

F-4

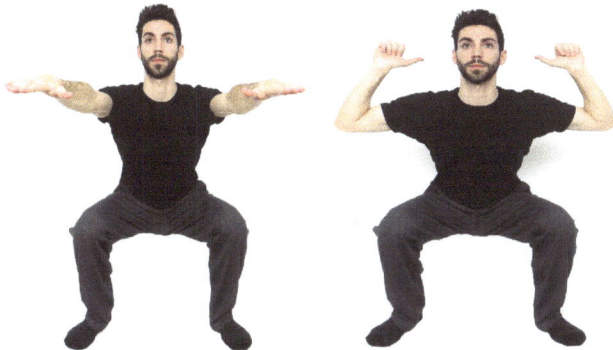

Start with your feet a little more than shoulder width apart and toes pointed slightly outwards. Squeeze your shoulder blades together and keep hands up and behind your head.

Stick your butt out, look up, keep spine fully straight and bend at your hips all the way down until knees are at about 90 degrees. As you move up, maintain your form and push outwards with your feet to further activate your gluteals.

F-5

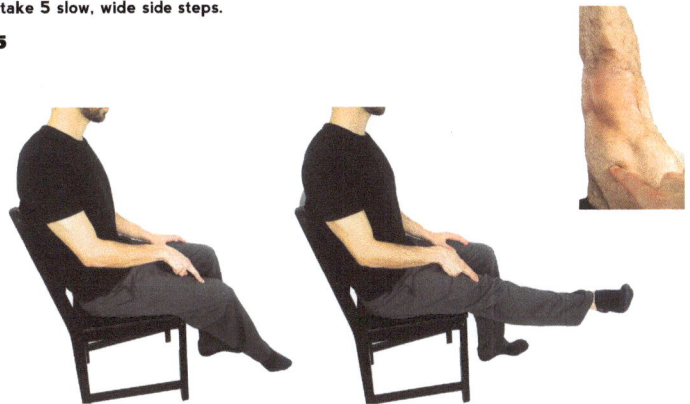

Sitting in a chair, slowly lift your foot with your toe pointed out. Squeeze your quadricep muscle once the leg is straight, hold for 2 seconds then slowly let it down.

Intesify the exercise by either wrapping a resistance band around the legs of the chair and the ankle, or by pushing firmly into the innermost quadricep muscle while you contract it.

203

F-6

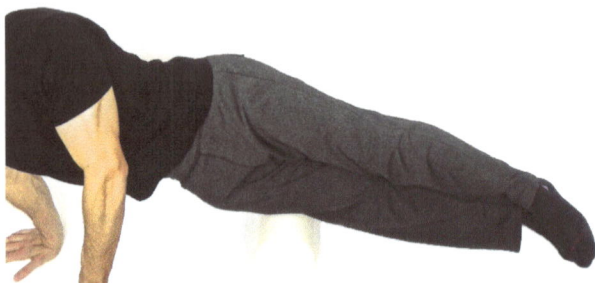

Lying on your side, place a foam roller under the side of your leg and use your arms to roll back and forth, guiding the pressure of the roller all along the length of your leg.

F-7

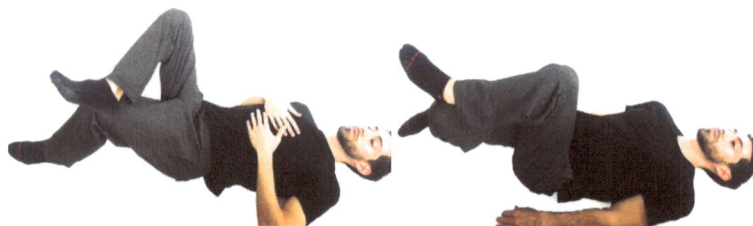

Lying on your back with knees bent, place the heel of one leg on the outside of the other leg and let that leg fall down and inwards.

Use the weight of the leg to stretch the hip further inwards.

F-8

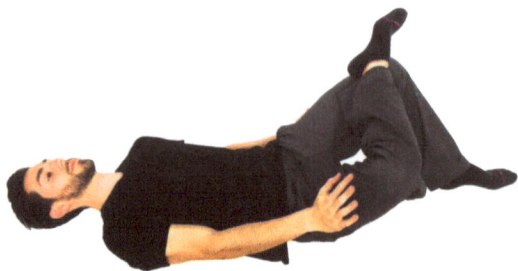

Lying on your back, place the outside of one ankle just above the other knee. Let the knee of the bent leg fall down toward the ground. Place gentle pressure on knee if needed. Hold for 30 seconds.

F-9

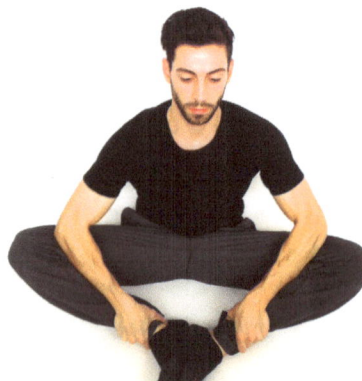

Sit and place the soles of your feet together. Then hold your ankles and use your elbows to push your knees down towards the ground.

F - 10

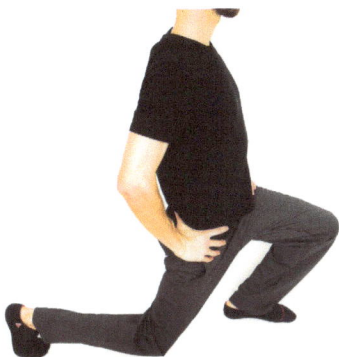

Take a large step forward with one leg, then slowly dip downwards and forwards into a lunge, leading with your pelvis. Hold for 30 seconds.

F - 11

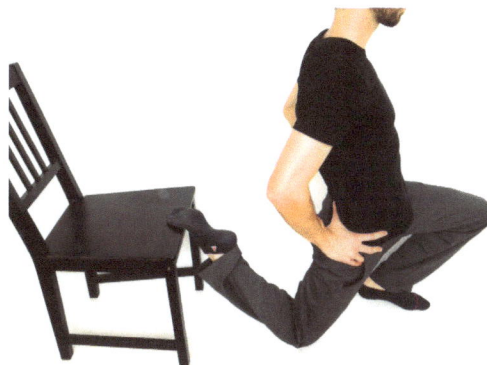

Place the top of your foot on a couch/chair, place your knee close to the base of the couch/chair, then put your other leg forward until the knee is bent to 90, then slowly dip down into a lunge and hold for 30 seconds.

F - 12

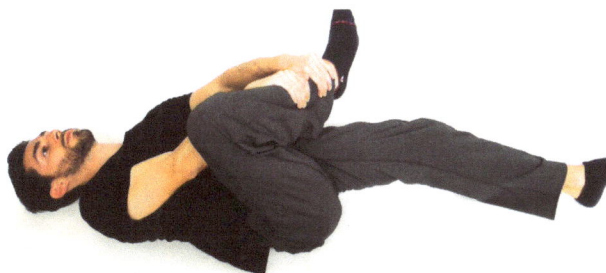

Lying on your back, bring your knee to your chest and a little across to the other side of your body. To intensify, pull the ankle of that leg up towards the opposite shoulder.

F - 13

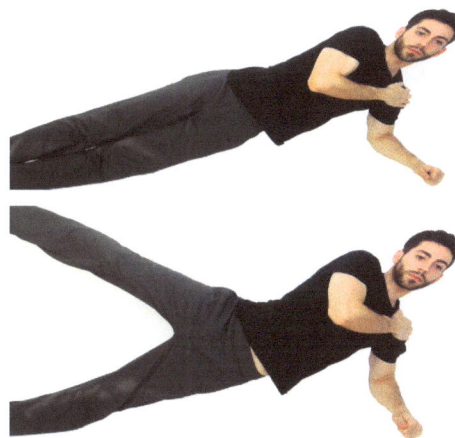

Lying on your side with your body straight and pelvis forward, lift your leg as high as you can. Keep your leg back and toe pointed up. Hold for 10 seconds. Repeat 3 times.

F - 14

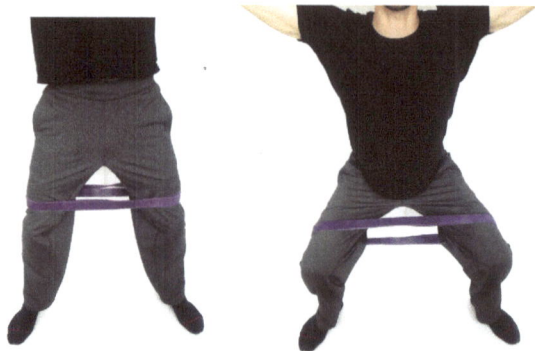

Double wrap a thick resistance band around your thighs just above your knees. Spread your legs a bit wider than shoulder width and point your toes slightly out.

Keep your head up, squeeze your shoulders together, keep your whole spine straight, squat slowly down, bending as far as you can through your hips, then slowly back up, holding your knees from moving inwards the whole time.

F - 15

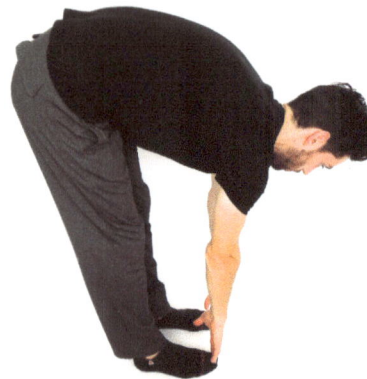

Keeping both legs together and knees straight, let your torso slowly relax forwards and down. For an extra stretch, hold your ankles and gently pull yourself down.

F - 16

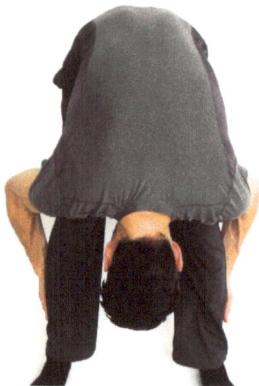

Standing with legs straight, bend your torso all the way down, relax your breath and gently pull your torso closer to your legs. Hold for 20 seconds.

F - 17

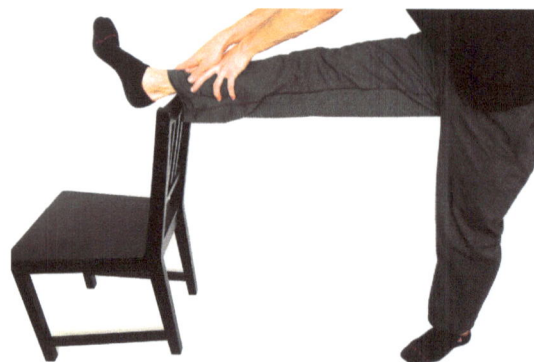

Bring your heel up on something roughly waist height. Keep your back straight and lower your torso down towards your foot.

F - 18

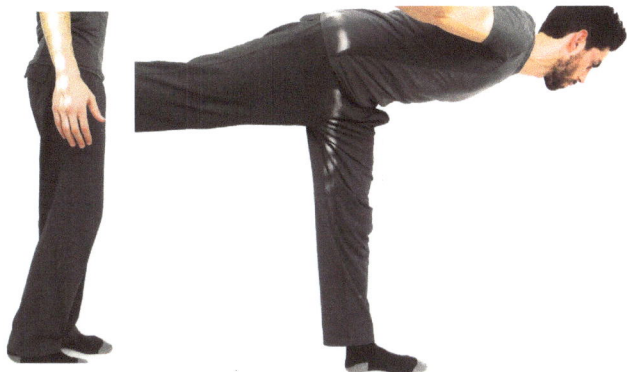

Balance on one leg, keeping it straight. Without allowing your pelvis to twist (keep it parallel to the floor), stick your arms out to the side and slowly bend down at the hips until 90 degrees. Slowly return to upright position. Repeat 10 times.

F - 19

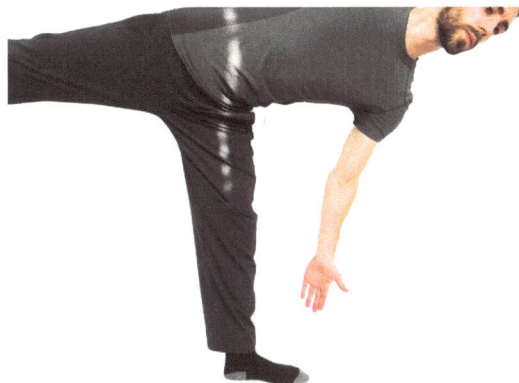

Advanced addition to exercise F - 18: Once down to 90 degrees, slowly twist the pelvis and arms, opening up as far as you can, return to position with pelvis level to the floor at a 90 degree bend, then slowly back upright. Do 10 reps.

F - 20

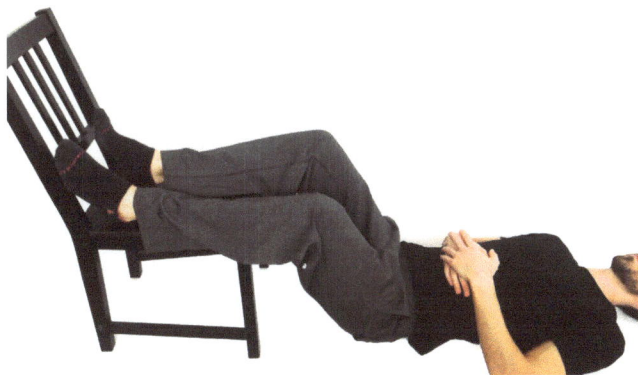

Lying on your back, put your legs up on a chair/couch up to the knee. Add or remove height until you feel a gentle decompression in your low back.

F - 21

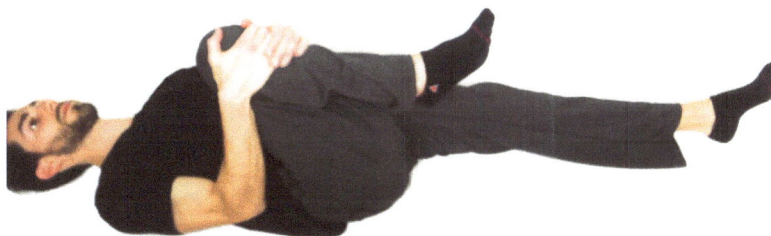

Lying on your back, bend one knee and use your arms to bring the leg right into your chest and hold. 25 seconds.

F - 22

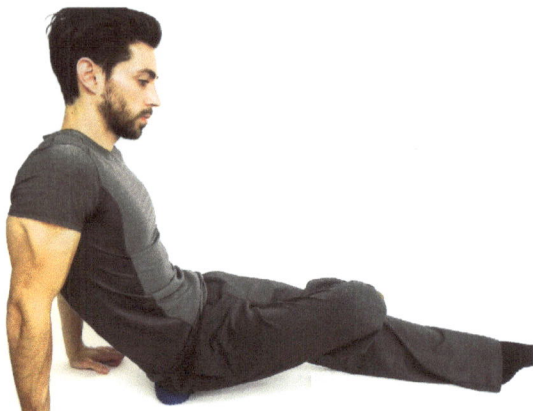

Sit one side of your bottom on the heated acuball, cross the leg into a figure 4 position. Hold the pressure on the tight areas. Gently move the knee up & down to intensify.

F - 23

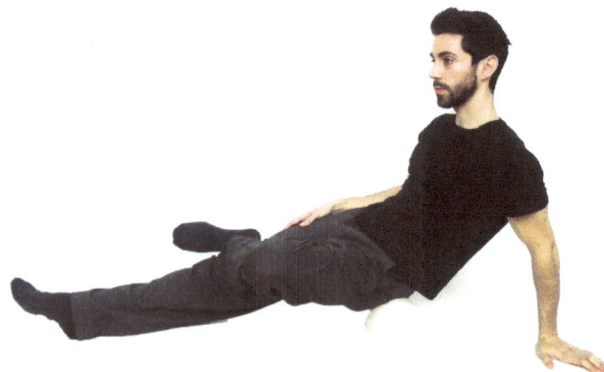

Start sitting with one cheek on a foam roller, cross that leg over the other in a figure 4 position and use your arms to roll your gluteal region over the roller.

F - 24

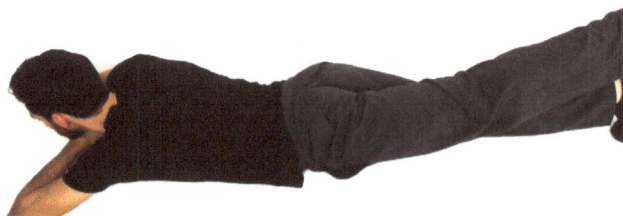

Lying face down, contract your core and raise one leg straight up. Ensure not to let your back bend. Do 30 lifts on each side.

F - 25

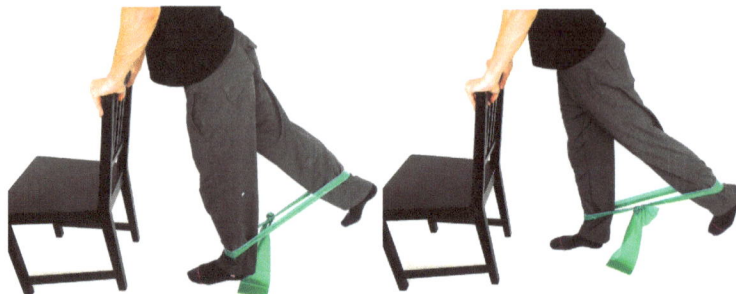

With a thick resistance band around both ankles, slowly extend one leg as far back as possible.

Hold a chair if needed. Perform 2 reps of 20 extensions on each side.

F - 26

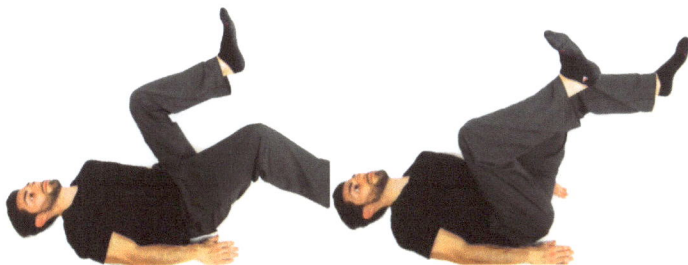

Lying on your back with your arms to your side, slowly cycle your legs as though you are riding an invisible bicycle.

Continue for 1-5 minutes.

F - 27

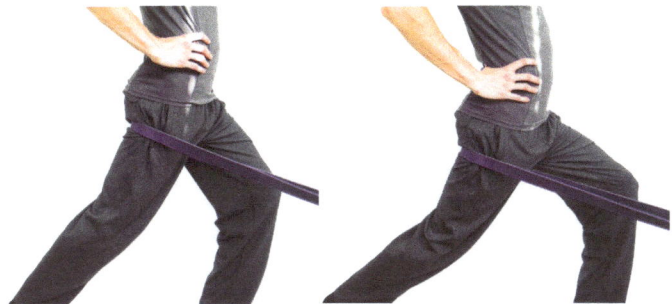

Fix a thick band to a sturdy structure in front of you and around your upper thigh. Slowly set down and back into a lunge. Hold for 3 seconds. Repeat 10 times on both sides.

F - 28

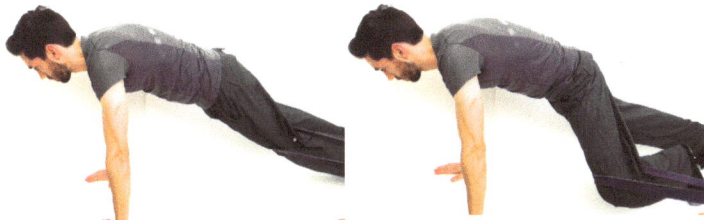

Fix a thick band to something sturdy. Wrap it around your thigh so it pulls outwards. Get in a pushup position.

Slowly pull thigh towards you and hold for 2 seconds. Repeat 10 times.

F - 29

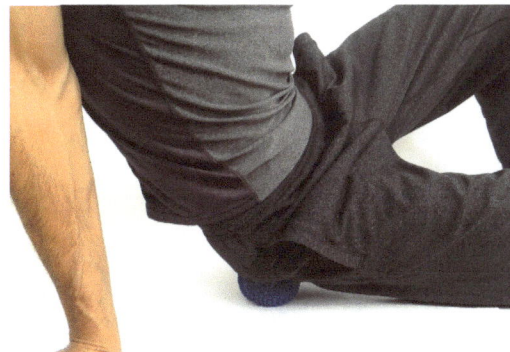

Either against a wall or sitting on a mat, slowly let your weight sink into the heated ball. Slowly rock your knee from side to side.

F - 30

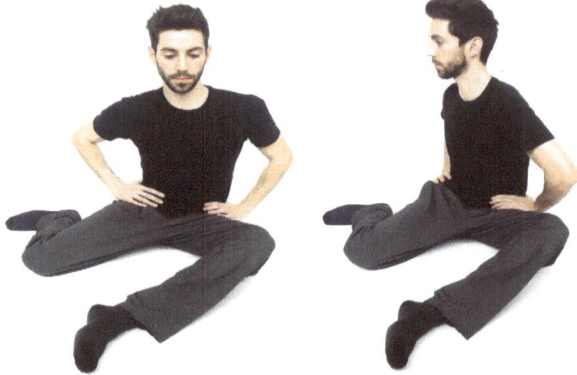

On the ground with legs as shown, move pelvis as upright and as forward as you can. Hold the position.

After 30 seconds, twist your torso 90 degrees to mobilize the hips in another direction.

F - 31

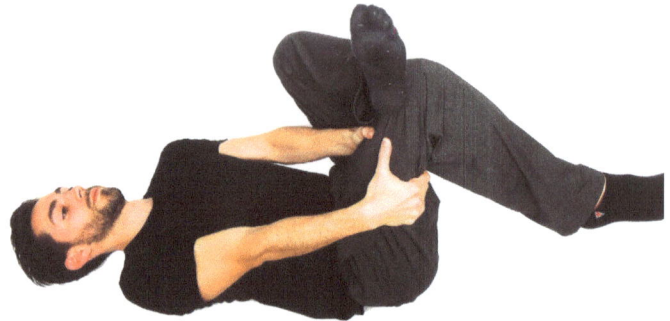

Lying on your back, bring your leg towards you, place the foot on the other thigh and relax hips. Pull in just under the knee and bring it towards you.

F - 32

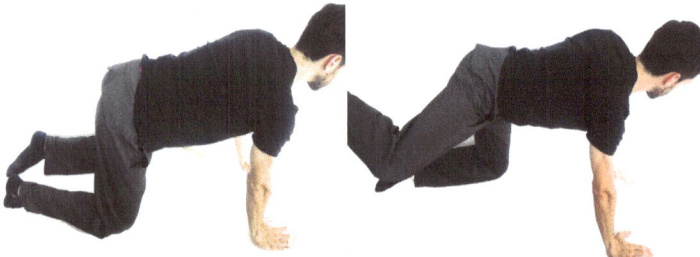

On your hands and knees, hold your pelvis square with the floor (don't let it tilt up) while lifting a leg as far up to the side as you can.

Hold for 30 seconds. Complete 3 sets of 10 reps for each leg.

F - 33

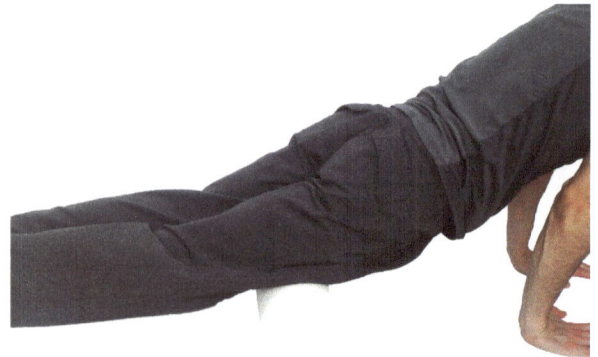

You can roll quads both at the same time, one at a time, or with legs crossed. Get in a push up position, place the roll under your thighs and roll back and forth.

F - 34

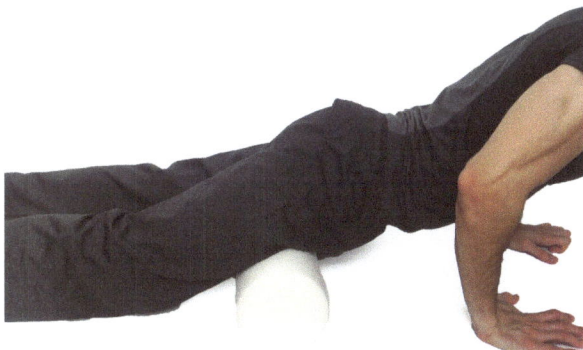

Start in a push up position, bring your torso up, place the foam roller under your inner thigh, point that foot all the way out to the side and push yourself back and forth.

F - 35

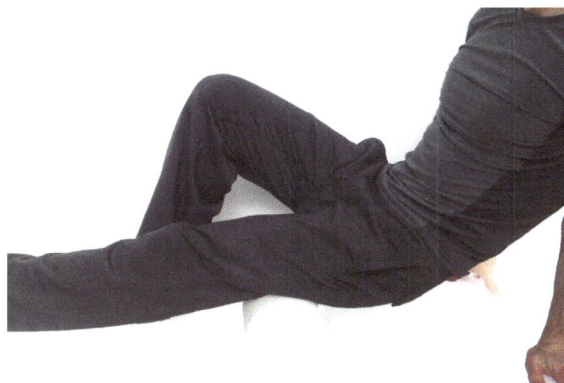

With one leg straight and the other foot on the ground, use your hands to move your body and roll your hamstrings back and forth over the foam roll. Alternatively cross one leg over the other, keep legs straight and roll.

G - 1

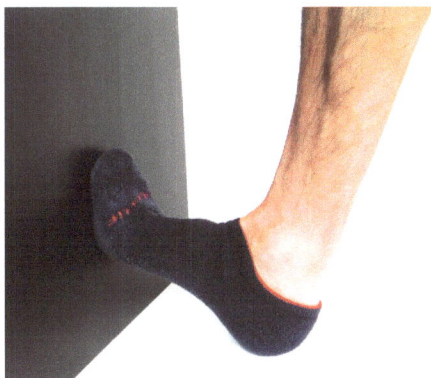

With a slightly bent knee, place your heel close to a wall with toes pointed up. Then slowly straighten your leg and move your body closer to the wall.

G - 2

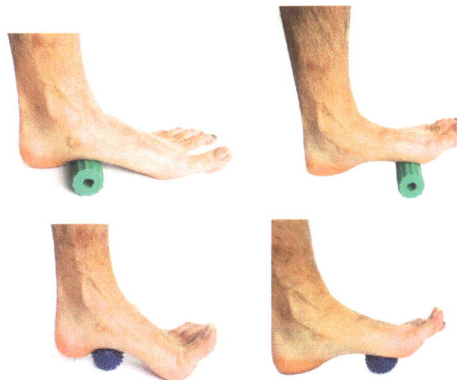

Slowly roll the bottom of your foot back and forth on the ball or roller. Apply pressure as tolerated.

G - 3

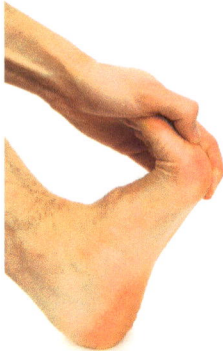

Lift all of your toes all the way up. If possible, also straighten your leg while you lift the toes.

G - 4

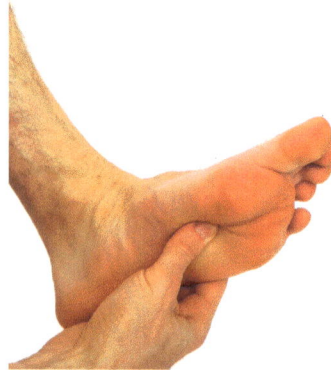

Hold all of your toes all the way up with one hand while you use the other to push firmly into the heel and swipe upwards slowly and deeply.

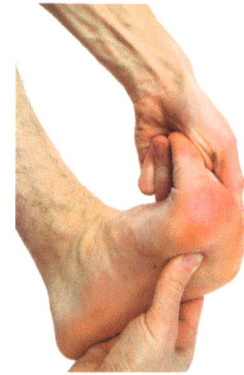

Work your way from the heel to toes, pushing in each spot while stretching the toes back. Repeat 10 times twice a day.

G - 5

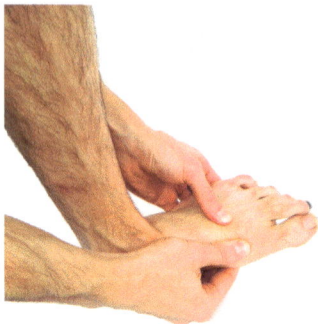

Grab the first long bone of your foot firmly. Grip the bone next to it firmly with the other hand.

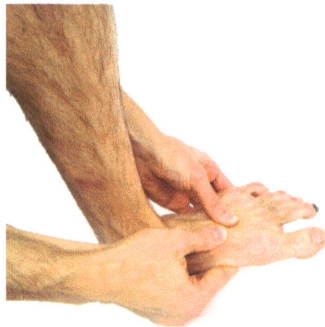

Move one up and one down, in opposite directions. Mobilize 10 times at each set of foot bones.

G - 6

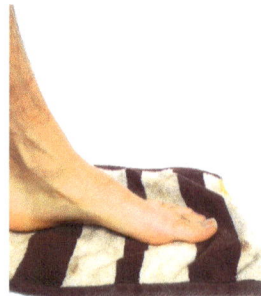

Squeeze your toes downwards to grip a towel on the floor enough to pick it up.

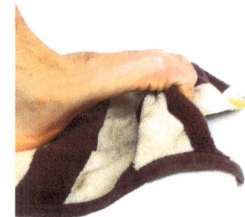

Aim to pick it up from the ball of your foot. Do 20 towel pickups per foot.

G - 7

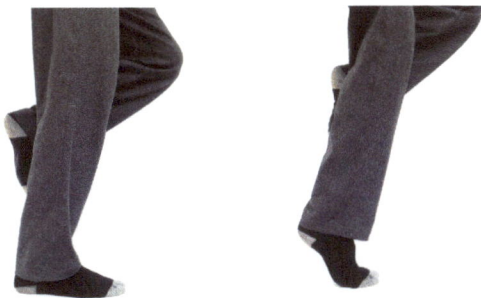

With one foot lifted up and held behind the other leg, slowly raise up onto your tip toes and then come slowly down.

Do thirty calf raises on each leg.

G - 8

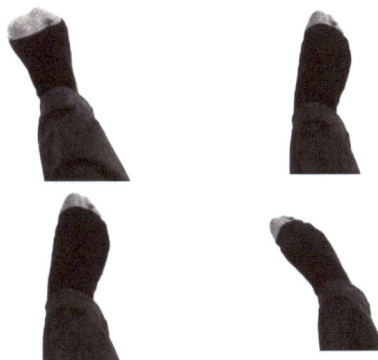

Imagine you are writing out each letter of the alphabet with your big toe. The bigger the better. Perform a full set of lower case and a full set of capital letters.

G - 9

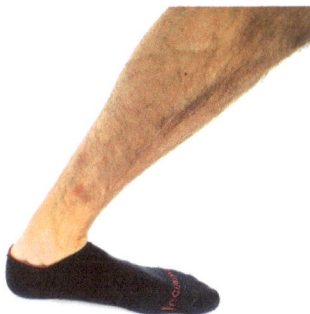

Step one leg three feet in front of the other, straighten your back leg fully and push your heel into the floor. 30 seconds.

G - 10

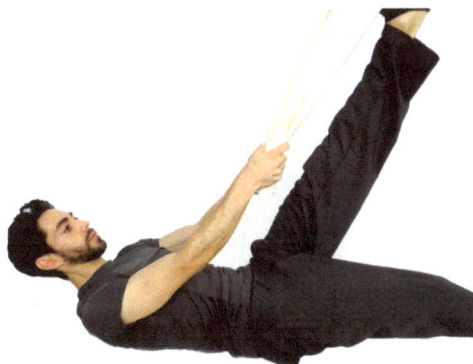

Lying on your back, wrap the middle of the towel around the ball of your foot, hold both ends, straighten and lift your leg and gently pull the towel towards you. Hold for 30 seconds on each side.

G - 11

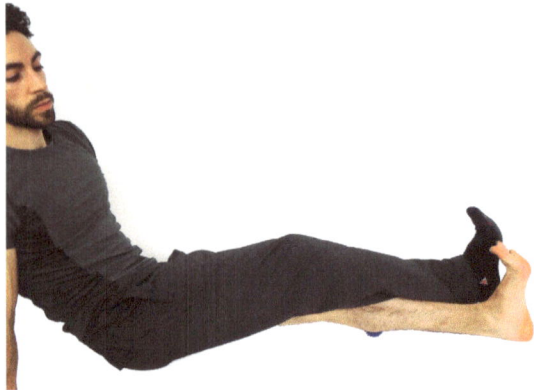

Crossing one leg over the other, use your hands to position the weight of your legs over the ball. Find a tender spot, hold pressure there and move your foot up and down.

G - 12

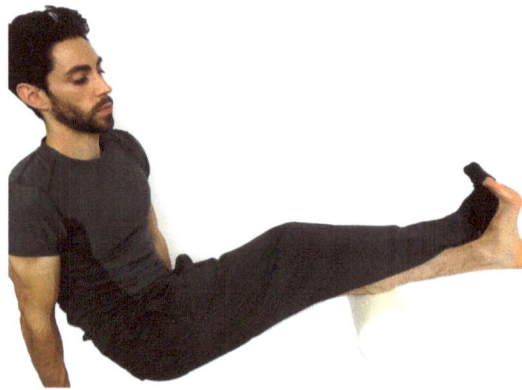

Crossing one leg over the other, use your hands to move yourself back and forth with the weight of your lower body on the foam roller.

G - 13

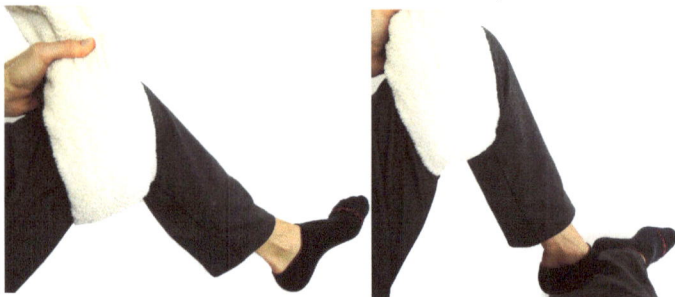

With the rolled up towel tucked right into the back of your knee.

Gently bend your leg and hold it at the end for 2 seconds. Repeat 8 times.

G - 14

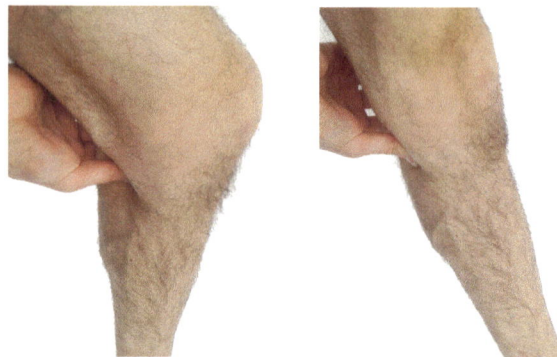

Find the tender spot on the inside, underside of your shin bone, right up at the top close to the knee.

Press firmly while you straighten your leg. Repeat 3 times.

G - 15

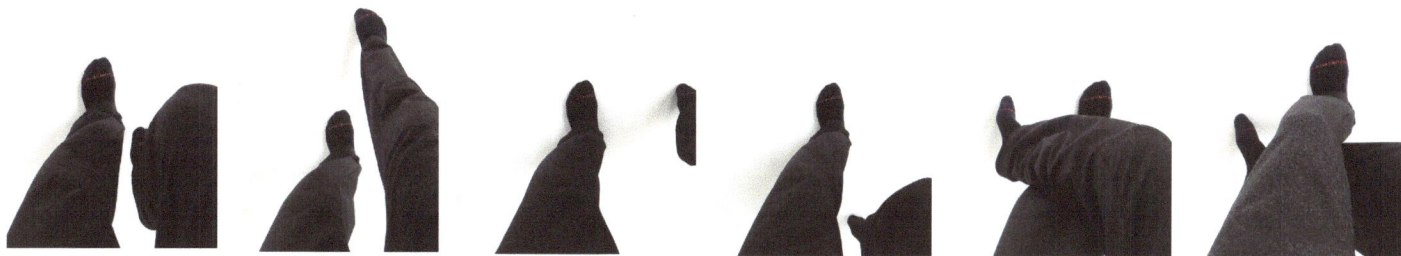

Balancing on the bad foot, reach as far away as you can to tap the toes of your other foot lightly in 5 points around you, complete a full circle. Hit each of the 4 cardinal points. Ensure to just tap the toe, do not put weight on the moving foot. As you get better, tap your toe farther away. Repeat 5 full rounds.

G - 16

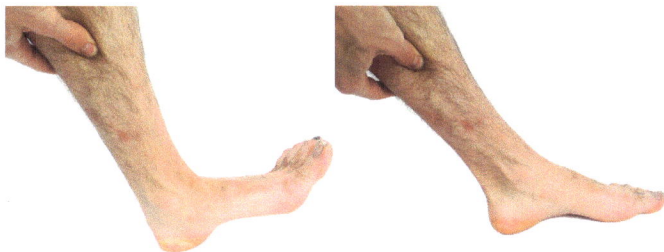

Roll off the inside edge of your shin bone, press and hold firmly on a spot while moving your foot slowly up and down.

Continue inching down the leg until you find the spot with the most tension. Do 6 repetitions of the move on that spot.

G - 17

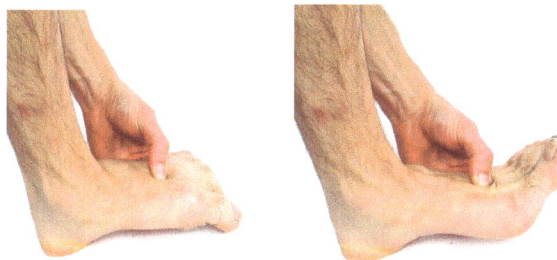

Squeeze firmly in-between each of the long bones in your foot and hold the pressure as you slowly raise and lower your toes.

Repeat several times in between each set of toes.

G - 18

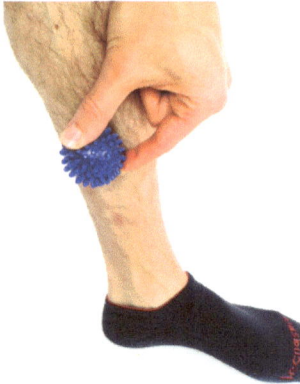

Push your foot into the ball, slowly run up the side of the foot right up to the big toe. When you feel tenderness, hold the pressure and raise the big toe up.

G - 19

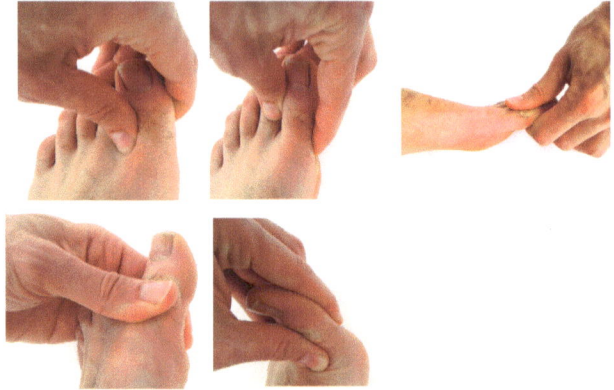

Gently pull the toe away from the foot, then to each side, up and down. Hold in each direction for 1 second. Repeat each 10 times.

G - 20

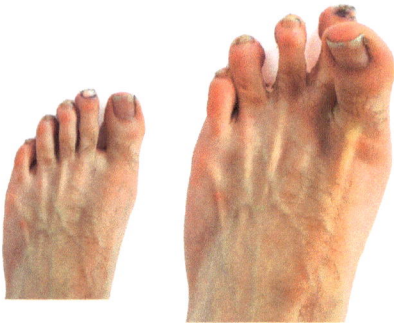

Starting one foot at a time, bare on the floor, push your forefoot into the ground and actively spread your toes as widely as possible, holding for 5 seconds. 15 reps.

G - 21

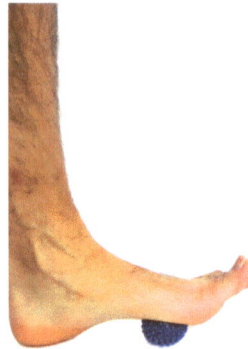

Using the middle part of the underside of your forefoot, pick a ball/marble off the floor, hold for 1 second then release. 30 reps with short rest breaks to prevent cramping.

G - 22

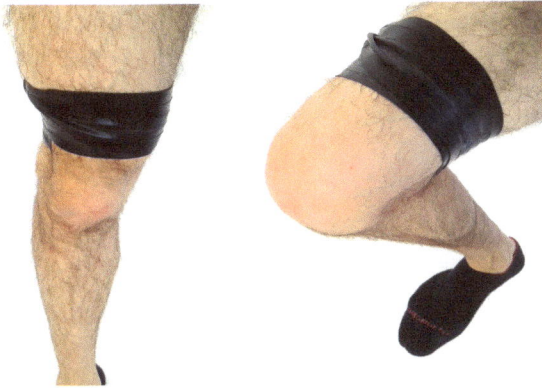

Cut a piece of bicycle tire inner tube or buy a VooDoo Band. Wrap tightly around leg 3 inches above the knee.

Slowly squat as deeply as comfortable. 6 reps.

G - 23

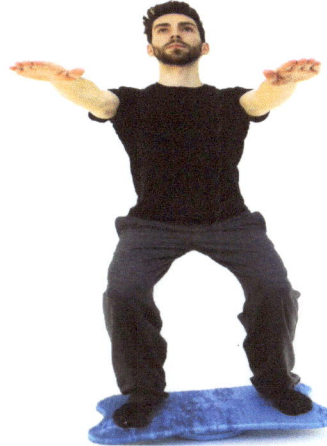

Keeping head tilted up, shoulders back and upright, bend knees slowly into a shallow squat and slowly back up. Maintain balance. 3 sets of 10 reps.

G - 24

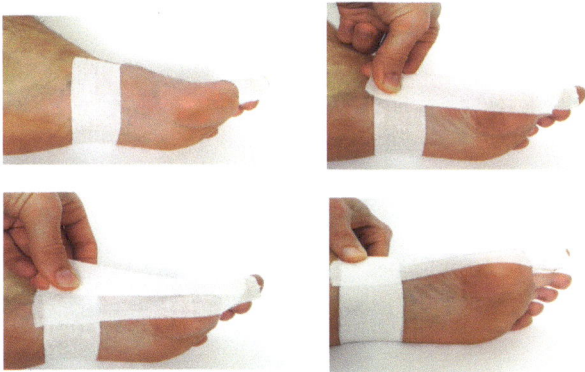

Apply a U-shaped 'anchor' around the bottom of the foot and a circle around the big toe. Add a strip from the toe to the anchor with enough tension to pull the big toe outwards.

Apply a second reinforcement strip from the toe to the anchor. Then reinforce both the toe circle and around the middle of the foot.

G - 25

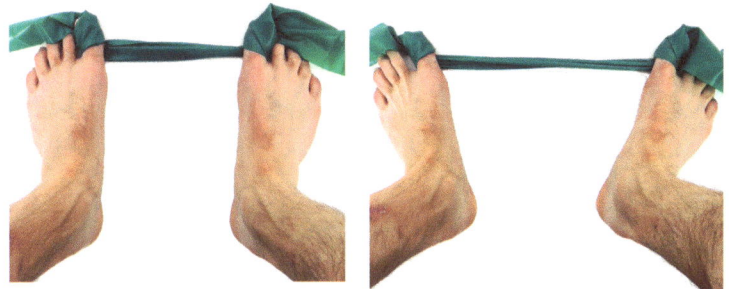

Wrap a light resistance band securely around both toes and pull until there is no slack.

Slowly turn both feet outwards to stretch the band and hold for 2 seconds. Repeat 20 times.

H - 1

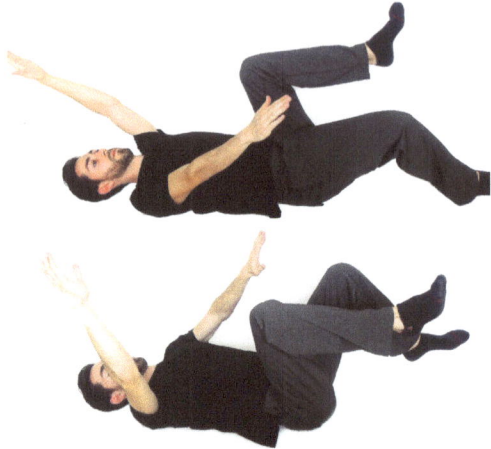

Lying on back with all limbs up, bring left arm halfway towards right leg, then alternate.

Move your limbs slowly. Work your way up to doing 6 sets of 1 minute.

H - 2

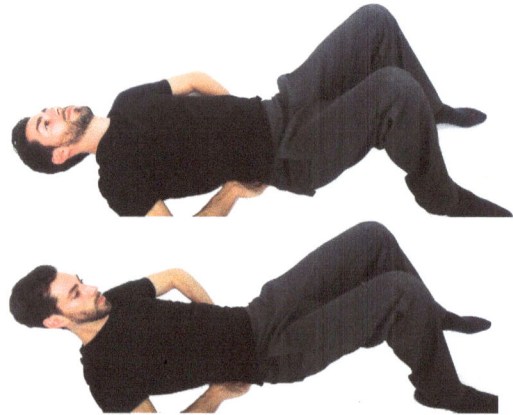

On your back with knees bent & hands under your low back, bring torso up just enough to get shoulders off the ground.

Squeeze abs to get a strong contraction. Slow, quality reps, (as many as you can) roughly 4 seconds each.

H - 3

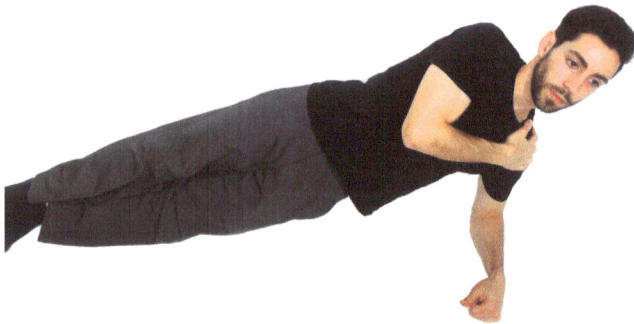

Holding yourself up onto your side with your forearm, bring your pelvis forward all the way until you are in a straight line. Hold yourself up & straight for 20 seconds. Repeat 4 times each side.

H - 4

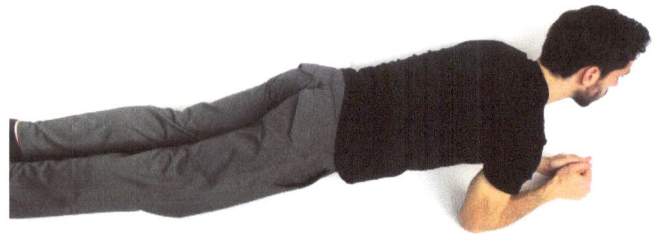

Holding yourself up with forearms shoulder width apart, bring your pelvis down until you are as straight as a plank. Hold for 20 seconds. Repeat 5 times.

H-5

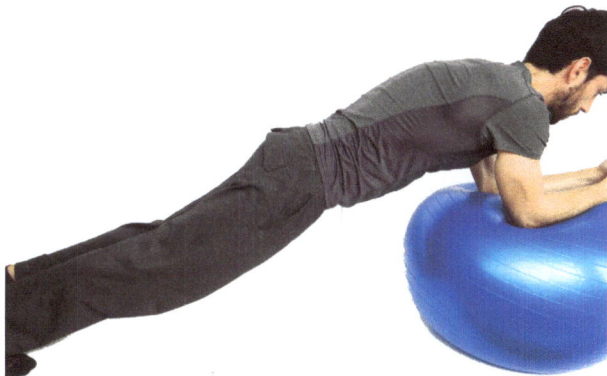

With hands clasped together and elbows flared out, move both forearms in a slow clockwise circle on the exercise ball. Your torso should remain still. Move VERY slowly and maintain good plank form. 3 sets 10 reps.

H-6

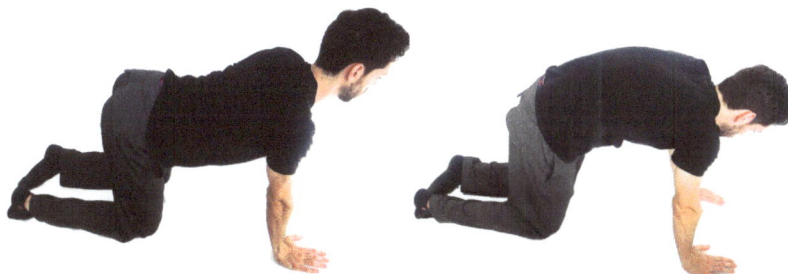

On hands & knees, breathe slowly in while arching your back all the upwards like a cat. Hold for 2 seconds.

Tilt pelvis forward & let your spine sink slowly down into a U shape. 20 reps.

H-7

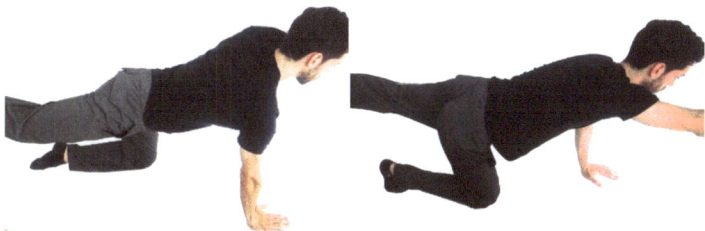

On hands & knees, keep spine straight & abs tight while slowly lifting the left arm and right leg simultaneously.

After 10 reps alternate limbs. Focus on coordination. 4 sets of 10 reps.

H-8

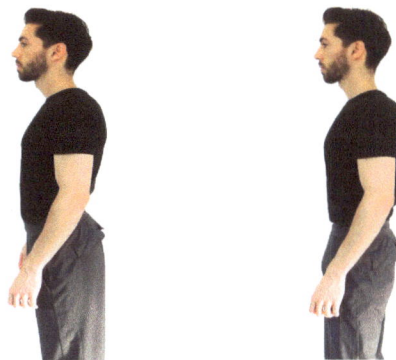

Moving only your pelvis, begin to slowly arch your back as far forward as it can go. Then your low back sink back towards the chair until flat.

Move your pelvis smoothly and slowly. Repeat 30 times.

H - 9

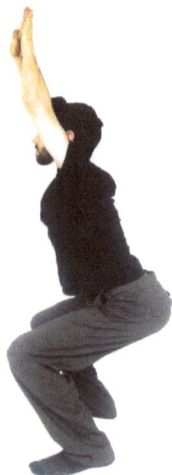

With your legs spread a touch more than shoulder width, toes pointed slightly outwards, head looking up, back straight and arms above your head with one hand on top of the other... Press your top hand firmly into the other and hold the pressure while you squat slowly right down to 90 degrees.

H - 10

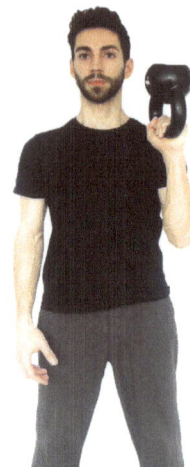

Hold a kettlebell upside down on one side at a time. Hold it above the collarbone and just in front of a shoulder. Hold your pelvis and core tight, keeping them stright and aligned. Hold for 1 minute on each side then repeat.

H - 11

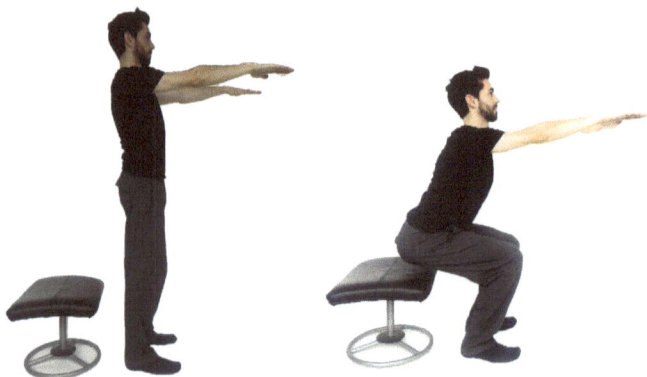

Stand a foot in front of a bucket or low bench. Hold your arms out straight in front of you. Slowly squat down, keeping your head up, chin tucked and shoulders back.

Keep your back straight and lower down until your bum touches the bench, but do not put your weight on it. Then slowly return to a standing position.

H - 12

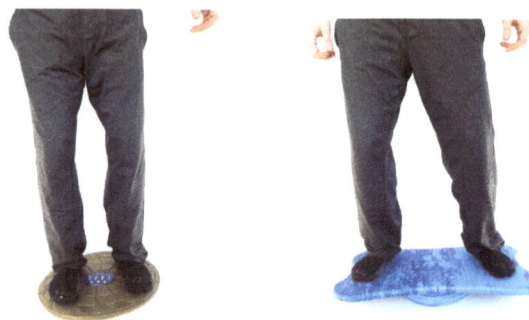

Balance with both feet on a wobble board. Keep your core engaged.

Slowly bend your knees slightly to increase the challange. Balance for 1 minute, then repeat a few times.

H - 13

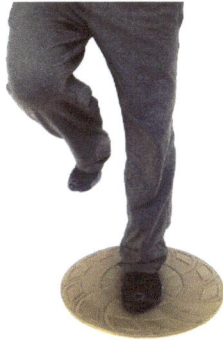

Stand on a wobble board balanced on one leg for as long as you can manage. Once you can stand for 1 minute without stumbling, move on to a more difficult board.

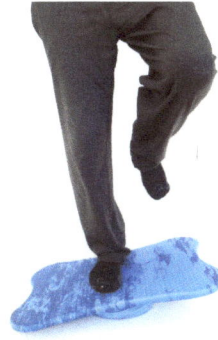

Moving up and down slowly increases the difficulty and the benefit.

H - 14

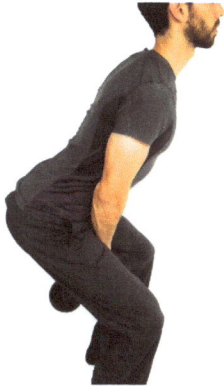

The kettlebell swing begins with the bell hanging between your legs, knees bent, shoulder blades together, head up and back straight. Let it swing gently backwards.

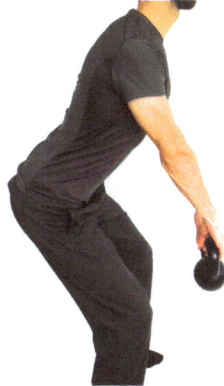

Thrust the bell forwards and up using your legs. Think of your arms as a rope in this exercise, the movement should all come from the hips. Squeeze your gluteals and push your feet slightly outwards as you thrust up.

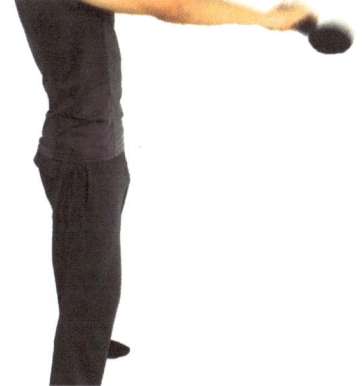

Let the bell swing up to about shoulder height and guide it as gravity swings it back down. Work towards timing it so it swings up and down uninterrupted.

APPENDIX

Appendix

Chemicals That Can Release Formaldehyde

Chemical	Synonym	CAS number
Formaldehyde	Formalin Methanal	50-00-0
Methylene glycol	Methanediol formalin formaldehyde monohydrate	463-57-0
Timonacic acid	thiazolidinecarboxylic acid, 1,3-thiazolidine-4-carboxylic acid	60731-25-1
(Phenylmethoxy)methanol	Benzylhemiformal benzyloxymethanol phenylmethoxymethanol Preventol D2	14548-60-8
7a-ethyldihydro-1H, 3H,5H-oxazolo[3,4-c]oxazole	Bioban CS-1246 ethyldihydrooxazolo[3,4-c]-oxazole 5-ethyl-1-aza-3,7-dioxa-bi-cyclo[3.3.0]octane	7747-35-5
Mixture of: 4-(2-nitrobutyl)morpholine and 4,4'-(2-ethyl-2-nitro-1,3-propanediyl)bismorpholine	Bioban P-1487 Mixture of: nitrobutylmorpholine and ethylnitrotrimethylenedimorpholine	37301-88-4 2224-44-4 1854-23-5
5-bromo-5-nitro-1,3-dioxane	Bromonitrodioxane Bronidox	30007-47-7
2-bromo-2-nitro-1,3-propanediol	Bromonitropropanediol Bronopol	52-51-7
N-(3-chloroallyl)hexamethylene-tetraminiumchloride	Chloroallylhexaminium chloride 3-chloroallyl hexaminiumchloride Dowicil 75 Dowicil 200 Quaternium 15	4080-31-3 cis(51229-78-8)

Chemicals That Can Release Formaldehyde Continued..

N-(1,3-bis(hydroxymethyl)2-5-dioxo-4-imidiazolidinyl)-N,N'-bis(hydroxymethyl)urea	Diazolidinyl urea tetramethylol hydanotin urea Germaben II Germall II	78491-02-8
Dimethoxymethane	Formal methylal	109-87-8
Formaldehyde, polymer with dimethyl-2,4-imidazolidinedione	Dimethylhydantoin formaldehyde resin DMHF	9065-13-8
N,N'-bis(hydroxymethyl)urea	Dimethylol urea dihydroxymethylurea dimethylurea urea formaldehyde	140-95-4
1,3-bis(hydroxymethyl)-5,5-dimethyl-2,4-imidazolidinedione	DMDM hydantoin dimethyloldimethylhydantoin 1,3-dimethylol-5,5-dimethylhydantoin DMDMH Glydant	6440-58-0
Mixture of: 1,3,5-triethylhexahydro-1,3,5 triazine and 1,3,5-triazine-1,3,5(2H,4H,6H) triethanol	Forcide 78 Mixture of: Triethylhexahydro s-triazine and trihydroxyethylhexahydro s-triazine	91925-30-3 7779-27-3 4719-04-4
1,3,5,7-tetraazatricyclo(3.3.1.1) decane	Hexamethylenetetramine hexamine methenamine Urotropine	100-97-0
2,4-imidazolidinedione	Hydantoin glycolylurea	461-72-3
N,N"-methylenebis(N'-(3-(hydroxymethyl)-2,5-dioxo-4-imidazolidinyl)urea)	Imidazolidinyl urea bis(methylolhydantoin urea) methane Euxyl K 200 Germall 115	39236-46-9

Chemicals That Can Release Formaldehyde Continued..

Hydroxymethly-5,5-dimethyl-2,4-imidazolidinedione	MDM hydantoin monomethyloldimethylhydanotin Dantoin 685 MDMH	27636-82-4
1-hydroxymethyl-5,5-dimethyl-2,4-imidazolidinedione		116-25-6
3-hydroxymethyl-5,5-dimethyl-2,4-imidazolidinedione		16228-00-5
3,3'-methylenebis(5-methyloxazolidine)	N,N'methylenebis(5-methyloxazolidine) Grotan OX	66204-44-2
2-chloro-N-(hydroxymethyl)-acetamide	N-methylolchloracetamide Grotan HD Parmetol K50 Preventol D3 Preventol D5	2832-19-1
2-(hydroxymethylamino)ethanol	N-methylolethanolamine	34375-28-5
Paraformaldehyde	Polyoxymethylene	30525-89-4
1,3,5-triazine-1,3,5(2H,4H,6H)-triethanol	Trihydroxyethylhexahydro s-triazine Grotan BK KM 200	4719-04-4
2-(hydroxymethyl)-2-nitro-1,3-propanediol	Tris(hydroxymethyl)nitromethane trimethylolnitromethane	126-11-4

Note: This list may not include all formaldehyde releasing chemicals

The above charts were adapted from: Fyvholm, MA, Andersen, P (1993): Identification of Formaldehyde Releasers and Occurrence of Formaldehyde and Formaldehyde Releasers in Registered Chemical Products.American Journal of Industrial Medicine 24(5):533-52.

References

Akpinar-Elci, M., A. Cimrin, and O. Elci. "Prevalence and Risk Factors of Occupational Asthma Among Hairdressers in Turkey." Journal of Occupational and Environmental Medicine 44 (2002): 585.

Alberta Health and Wellness. "Health Standards and Guidelines for Barbering and Hairstyling." Government of Alberta (2002): 1 - 5. Accessed June 2015. http://www.health.alberta.ca/documents/Standards-Barber-Hairstyling.pdf

Baan, Robert, Kurt Straif, Yann Grosse, Beatrice Secretan, Fatiha El Ghissassi, Veronique Bouvard, Lamia Benbrahim-Tallaa, and Vincent Cogliano. "Carcinogenicity of Some Aromatic Amines, Organic Dyes, and Related Exposures." The Lancet Oncology 9 (2008)

Bain, G. I. and N. A. Wallwork. "Percutaneous A1 Pulley Release a Clinical Study." Hand Surgery 4(1999)

Balch, Phyllis. Prescription for Nutritional Healing, 4th ed. New York: Avery, 2006.

Baste V., B. E. Moen, T. Riise, B. E. Hollund, and N. J. Øyen. "Infertility and Spontaneous Abortion Among Female Hairdressers: The Hordaland Health Study." Occupational and Environmental Medicine 50 (2008): 1371-1377.

Bilchik, T. R. "A Review of Nonvalidated and Complementary Therapies for Cluster Headache." Current Pain Headache Reports, 8 (2004): 157-61.

Brown, Nellie. J. Health Hazard Manual for Cosmetologists, Hairdressers, Beauticians and Barbers. New York: Cornell University, 1987.

Bruce P. Bernard. "Musculoskeletal Disorders and Workplace Factors." National Institute for Occupational Safety and Health (1997).

Burstein, Rami, and Moshe Jakubowski. "Unitary Hypothesis for Multiple Triggers of Pain and Strain of Migraine." Journal of Comparative Neurology 14 (2005): 9-14.

Ding, C., F. Cicuttini, F. Scott, C. Boon, and G. Jones. "Association of Prevalent and Incident Knee Cartilage Defects with Loss of Tibial and Patellar Cartilage: A Longitudinal Study." Arthritis & Rheumatism 52 (2005): 3918–3927. doi: 10.1002/art.21474

Earl, J. E., and A. Z. Hoch. "A Proximal Strengthening Program Improves Pain, Function, and Biomechanics in Women with Patellofemoral Pain Syndrome." American Journal of Sports Medicine 39 (2011): 154–63.

Fowler J. R., and M. E. Baratz. "Percutaneous trigger finger release." Journal of Hand Surgery American Volume 38 (2013): 2005.

Haldeman S and S. Degenais. "Choosing a Treatment for Cervicogenic Headache: When? What? How much?." The Spine Journal 2010; 10: 169-71.

International Headache Society. "The International Classification of Headache Disorders." Cephalgia 1 (2004): 1-151.

Kersemaekers W. M., N. Roeleveld, and G. A. Zielhuis. "Reproductive Disorders Due to Chemical Exposure Among Hairdressers." Scandinavian Journal of Work, Environment and Health 21 (1995): 325 – 334.

Khayambashi K, Z. Mohammadkhani, K. Ghaznavi, M. A. Lyle, and C. M. Powers. "The Effects of Isolated Hip Abductor and External Rotator Muscle Strengthening on Pain, Health Status, and Hip Strength in Females with Patellofemoral Pain: a Randomized Controlled Trial." Journal of Orthopaedic and Sports Physical Therapy 42 (2012): 22

Marie-Louise Lind. "Hairdressers –Hand Eczema, Hair Dyes and Hand Protection," THE DEPARTMENT OF WORK AND HEALTH, National Institute for Working Life, Stockholm, Sweden, 2006.

Mishra S. R., A. k Gaur, M. M. Choudhary, and J. Ramesh. "Percutaneous A1 Pulley Release by the Tip of a 20-g Hypodermic Needle Before Open Surgical Procedure in Trigger Finger Management." Techniques in Hand Upper Extremity Surgery 17 (2013): 112.

Moscato, G., G. Pala, L. Perfetti, M. Frascaroli, and P. Pignatti. "Clinical and Inflammatory Features of Occupational Asthma Caused by Persulphate Salts in Comparison with Asthma Associated with Occupational Rhinitis." Allergy 65 (2010): 784-790. doi: 10.1111/j.1398- 9995.2009.02288.x

Mounier-Geyssant, E., V. Oury, L. Mouchot, C. Paris, and D. Zmirou-Navier. "Exposure of Hairdressing Apprentices to Airborne Hazardous Substances." Environmental Health: A Global Access Science Source 5 (2006)

Mussi, Gisele and Nelson Gouveia. "Prevalence of Work-Related Musculoskeletal Disorders in Brazilian Hairdressers." Occupational Medicine 58 (2008): 367-369. doi: 10.1093/occmed/kqn047

Nicholson, G. and J. Gaston. "Cervical Headache." Journal of Orthopaedic & Sports Physical Therapy 31 (2001): 184-193.

O'Connor, Francis G. Sports Medicine: Just The Facts. Location: McGraw-Hill, 2005.

Occupational Safety and Health Administration. "Hair Salons: Facts About Formaldehyde in Hair Products; Formaldehyde in Your Products." Accessed March 16, 2014. https://www.osha.gov/SLTC/hairsalons/formaldehyde_in_products.html

Peters, C., M. Harling, and M. Dulon. "Fertility Disorders and Pregnancy Complications in Hairdressers – A Systematic Review." Journal of Occupational Medicine and Toxicology 5 (2010)

Peters-Veluthamaningal C., J. C. Winters, K. H. Groenier, and B. M Jong. "Corticosteroid Injections Effective for Trigger Finger in Adults in General Practice: A Double-Blinded Randomised Placebo Controlled Trial." Annals of the Rheumatic Diseases 67 (2008): 1262.

Pierce, J. S., A. Abelmann, L. J. Spicer, R. E. Adams, M. E., Glynn, K. Neier, B. L. Finley, and S. H. Gaggney. "Characterization of Formaldehyde Exposure Resulting from the Use of Four Professional Hair Straightening Products." Journal of Occupational Environmental Hygiene 8 (2011): page range. DOI:10.1080/15459624.2011.626259

Stefanik, J. J., A. Guermazi, Y. Zhu, A. C. Zumwalt, K. D. Gross, M. Clancy, J. A. Lynch, N. A. Segal, C. E. Lewis, F. W. Roemer, C. M. Powers, and D. T. Felson. "Quadriceps Weakness, Patella Alta, and Structural Features of Patellofemoral Osteoarthritis." Arthritis Care and Research 63 (2011): 1391–1397. doi: 10.1002/acr.20528

Sun-Edelstein, Christina, and Alexander Mauskop. "Foods and Supplements in the Management of Migraine Headaches." The Clinical Journal of Pain 25, (2009): 446-52.

Trinh K.V., N. Graham, A. R. Gross, C. H. Goldsmith, E. Wang, I. D. Cameron, T. Kay., and Cervical Overview Group. Acupuncture for Neck Disorders. Cochrane Database Systematic Reviews 2006, CD004870.

Turowski, G. A., P. D. Zdankiewicz, and J. G. Thomson. "The Results of Surgical Treatment of Trigger Finger." Journal of Hand Surgery American Volume 22 (1997): 145.

Vizniak, Nikita A., and Michael A. Carnes. Quick Reference Clinical Chiropractic Conditions Manual. Location: Professional Health Systems, 2004.

Wang J., J. G. Zhao, and C. C. Liang. "Percutaneous Release, Open Surgery, or Corticosteroid Injection, Which is the Best Treatment Method for Trigger Digits?." Clinical Orthopaedics and Related Research 471 (2013): 1879.

Safety Information and Disclaimer: The information in this book is not intended as a substitute for professional advice from doctors and other relevant experts. The advice on physical or mental health, fitness and exercise, diet and supplementation and drugs and surgery are meant to help you make informed decisions on your health, but are not meant for self-diagnosis. If you suspect you have an injury or medical condition, you should seek the approval of your doctor or therapist before taking on new exercises or therapies. Do no attempt to self-treat serious or long-term problems without first consulting a qualified health-care practitioner. If you are currently undergoing a prescribed course of medical or pharmacological treatment, do not self-treat or make any dietary (herb, supplements or foods) changes until approved by the professionals administering your medical treatment. The author is not engaged in rendering professional advice or services to the individual reader. The author takes no responsibility for injury to persons or property that results from the advice given in this book.

About The Author

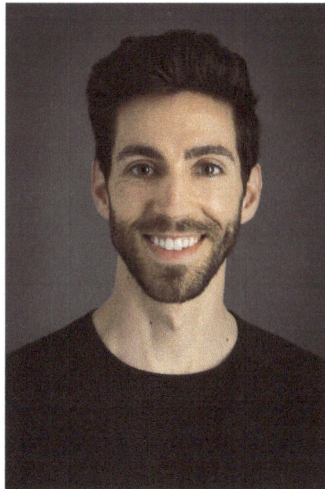

Jonas is a chiropractor and consultant in Toronto, Canada.